Neuroradiology: Updates in Brain Imaging

Editors

SHIRA E. SLASKY
JACQUELINE A. BELLO

RADIOLOGIC CLINICS OF NORTH AMERICA

www.radiologic.theclinics.com

Consulting Editor
FRANK H. MILLER

November 2019 • Volume 57 • Number 6

ELSEVIER

1600 John F. Kennedy Boulevard • Suite 1800 • Philadelphia, Pennsylvania, 19103-2899

http://www.theclinics.com

RADIOLOGIC CLINICS OF NORTH AMERICA Volume 57, Number 6
November 2019 ISSN 0033-8389, ISBN 13: 978-0-323-71046-6

Editor: John Vassallo (j.vassallo@elsevier.com)
Developmental Editor: Donald Mumford

Radiologic Clinics of North America (ISSN 0033-8389) is published bimonthly by Elsevier Inc., 360 Park Avenue South, New York, NY 10010-1710. Months of issue are January, March, May, July, September, and November. Periodicals postage paid at New York, NY and additional mailing offices. Subscription prices are USD 508 per year for US individuals, USD 933 per year for US institutions, USD 100 per year for US students and residents, USD 594 per year for Canadian individuals, USD 1193 per year for Canadian institutions, USD 683 per year for international individuals, USD 1193 per year for international institutions, and USD 315 per year for Canadian and international students/residents. To receive student and resident rate, orders must be accompanied by name of affiliated institution, date of term and the signature of program/residency coordinatior on institution letterhead. Orders will be billed at individual rate until proof of status is received. Foreign air speed delivery is included in all *Clinics* subscription prices. All prices are subject to change without notice. **POSTMASTER:** Send address changes to *Radiologic Clinics of North America*, Elsevier Health Sciences Division, Subscription Customer Service, 3251 Riverport Lane, Maryland Heights, MO63043. **Customer Service: Telephone: 1-800-654-2452** (U.S. and Canada); **1-314-447-8871** (outside U.S. and Canada). **Fax: 1-314-447-8029. E-mail: journalscustomerservice-usa@elsevier.com (for print support); journalsonlinesupport-usa@elsevier.com (for online support)**.

Reprints. For copies of 100 or more of articles in this publication, please contact the Commercial Reprints Department, Elsevier Inc., 360 Park Avenue South, New York, New York 10010-1710. Tel.: +1-212-633-3874; Fax: +1-212-633-3820; E-mail: reprints@elsevier.com.

Radiologic Clinics of North America also published in Greek Paschalidis Medical Publications, Athens, Greece.

Radiologic Clinics of North America is covered in *MEDLINE/PubMed (Index Medicus), EMBASE/Excerpta Medica, Current Contents/Life Sciences, Current Contents/Clinical Medicine, RSNA Index to Imaging Literature, BIOSIS, Science Citation Index,* and *ISI/BIOMED.*

Contributors

CONSULTING EDITOR

FRANK H. MILLER, MD, FACR
Lee F. Rogers MD Professor of Medical
Education, Chief, Body Imaging Section and
Fellowship Program, Medical Director, MRI,
Department of Radiology, Northwestern
Memorial Hospital, Northwestern University
Feinberg School of Medicine, Chicago, Illinois

EDITORS

SHIRA E. SLASKY, MD
Assistant Professor, Department of Radiology,
Division of Neuroradiology, Albert Einstein
College of Medicine, Montefiore Medical
Center, Bronx, New York

JACQUELINE A. BELLO, MD, FACR
Professor of Clinical Radiology and
Neurosurgery, Director of Neuroradiology,
Division of Neuroradiology, Department of
Radiology, Albert Einstein College of Medicine,
Montefiore Medical Center, Bronx, New York

AUTHORS

BEHNAM BADIE, MD
Division Chief and Professor, Department of
Neurosurgery, City of Hope National Cancer
Center, Los Angeles, California

JACQUELINE A. BELLO, MD, FACR
Professor of Clinical Radiology and
Neurosurgery, Director of Neuroradiology,
Division of Neuroradiology, Department of
Radiology, Albert Einstein College of Medicine,
Montefiore Medical Center, Bronx, New York

JUDAH BURNS, MD
Associate Professor of Radiology, Albert
Einstein College of Medicine, Montefiore
Medical Center, Bronx, New York

ABBAS CHAUDHRY, PharmD
Post-doctoral Fellow, Department of
Diagnostic Radiology, City of Hope National
Cancer Center, Los Angeles, California

AMMAR A. CHAUDHRY, MD
Director, Precision Imaging Lab, Associate
Director of Imaging Informatics Research,
Assistant Professor, Department of Diagnostic
Radiology, City of Hope National Cancer
Center, Los Angeles, California

MELISSA M. CHEN, MD
Assistant Professor, Department of Diagnostic
Radiology, Division of Diagnostic Imaging, The
University of Texas MD Anderson Cancer
Center, Houston, Texas

MIKE CHEN, MD, PhD
Associate Professor, Department of
Neurosurgery, City of Hope National Cancer
Center, Los Angeles, California

GLORIA C. CHIANG, MD
Associate Professor, Department of Radiology,
Division of Neuroradiology, Weill Cornell
Medical Center, New York, New York

EDWARD J. EBANI, MD
Diagnostic Radiology Resident, Department of
Radiology, Weill Cornell Medical Center, New
York, New York

KAREM GHARZEDDINE, MD
Assistant Attending, Department of Radiology, Memorial Sloan-Kettering Cancer Center, New York, New York

MARYAM GUL, MD
Assistant Professor, Department of Diagnostic Radiology, City of Hope National Cancer Center, Los Angeles, California

AJAY GUPTA, MD, MS
Associate Professor of Radiology and Neuroscience, Vice Chair for Research, Department of Radiology, Weill Cornell Medicine, New York, New York

VAIOS HATZOGLOU, MD
Associate Attending, Assistant Professor, Department of Radiology, Memorial Sloan-Kettering Cancer Center, Weill Medical College of Cornell University, New York, New York

JEREMY J. HEIT, MD, PhD
Department of Radiology, Division of Neuroimaging and Neurointervention, Stanford Healthcare, Stanford, California

STEVEN HETTS, MD
Professor of Radiology and Biomedical Imaging, Division of Neurointerventional Radiology, University of California, San Francisco, San Francisco, California

ANDREI I. HOLODNY, MD, PhD (hon), FACR
Chief of the Neuroradiology Service, Director of the Functional MRI Laboratory, Professor, Department of Radiology, Memorial Sloan-Kettering Cancer Center, Weill Medical College of Cornell University, Professor of Neuroscience, Weill Cornell Graduate School of Medical Sciences, New York, New York

CAMILO JAIMES, MD
Department of Radiology, Staff Neuroradiologist, Boston Children's Hospital, Instructor of Radiology, Harvard Medical School, Boston, Massachusetts

RAHUL JANDIAL, MD, PhD
Associate Professor, Department of Neurosurgery, City of Hope National Cancer Center, Los Angeles, California

RAJKAMAL KHANGURA, MD
Department of Radiology and Biomedical Imaging, Division of Neurointerventional Radiology, University of California, San Francisco, San Francisco, California

ASHLEY KNIGHT-GREENFIELD, MD
Department of Radiology, Weill Cornell Medicine, New York, New York

KELLY K. KOELLER, MD
Department of Radiology, Mayo Clinic Minnesota, Rochester, Minnesota

ALEX LEVITT, MD
Attending Neuroradiologist, Jacobi Medical Center, Albert Einstein College of Medicine, Bronx, New York

CHRISTIE M. MALAYIL LINCOLN, MD
Assistant Professor, Department of Radiology, Baylor College of Medicine, Houston, Texas

ALICIA MENG, MD
Neuroradiology Fellow, Department of Radiology, Weill Cornell Medical Center, New York, New York

SOHAIB NAIM, BSc
Research Associate, Department of Diagnostic Radiology, City of Hope National Cancer Center, Los Angeles, California

JOEL JOSE QUITLONG NARIO, BS
Department of Radiology, Weill Cornell Medicine, New York, New York

TINA YOUNG POUSSAINT, MD, FACR
Professor, Department of Radiology, Boston Children's Hospital, Harvard Medical School, Director, PBTC Neuroimaging Center, Chair, Institutional Review Board, Boston, Massachusetts

JAVIER M. ROMERO, MD
Associate Professor, Department of Neuroradiology, Massachusetts General Hospital, Harvard Medical School, Boston, Massachusetts

PAMELA W. SCHAEFER, MD
Professor, Department of Neuroradiology, Massachusetts General Hospital, Harvard Medical School, Boston, Massachusetts

ROBERT Y. SHIH, MD
Department of Radiology, Uniformed Services
University, Bethesda, Maryland

SHIRA E. SLASKY, MD
Assistant Professor, Department of Radiology,
Division of Neuroradiology, Albert Einstein
College of Medicine, Montefiore Medical
Center, Bronx, New York

JAE W. SONG, MD, MS
Assistant Professor, Department of Radiology,
Division of Neuroradiology, University of
Pennsylvania, Philadelphia, Pennsylvania

JENNIFER E. SOUN, MD
Assistant Professor, Department of
Radiological Sciences, University of California,
Irvine, Orange, California

SARA B. STRAUSS, MD
Neuroradiology Fellow, Department of
Radiology, Weill Cornell Medical Center,
New York, New York

ERIC S. SUSSMAN, MD
Department of Radiology, Division of
Neuroimaging and Neurointervention,
Department of Neurosurgery, Stanford
Healthcare, Stanford, California

KEVIN YUQI WANG, MD
Resident, Department of Radiology, Baylor
College of Medicine, Houston, Texas

MAX WINTERMARK, MD
Department of Radiology, Division of
Neuroimaging and Neurointervention, Stanford
Healthcare, Stanford, California

ROBERT J. YOUNG, MD
Director, Brain imaging, Director,
Neuroradiology Research, Associate
Attending, Neuroradiology Service,
Department of Radiology, Memorial Sloan
Kettering Cancer Center, New York, New York

RICHARD ZAMPOLIN, MD
Assistant Professor of Radiology, Albert
Einstein College of Medicine, Montefiore
Medical Center, Bronx, New York

Contents

This article reviews the current state of imaging for acute ischemic stroke. Protocolized imaging acquisition using computed tomography in conjunction with coordinated stroke care allows for rapid diagnosis and prompt revascularization. Following the initial evidence to support endovascular therapy for large-vessel occlusion, published between 2014 and 2015, there are now guidelines supporting treatment up to 24 hours after time of onset of symptoms. Neuroimaging remains a central component in diagnosing acute stroke and potentially excluding patients from stroke treatment, as outlined in this article.

Acute stroke is a leading cause of morbidity and mortality in the United States. Acute ischemic strokes have been classified according to The Trial of Org 10172 in Acute Stroke Treatment (TOAST) classification system, and this system aids in proper management. Nearly every patient who presents to a hospital with acute stroke symptoms has some form of emergent imaging. As such, imaging plays an important role in early diagnosis and management. This article reviews the imaging patterns of acute strokes, and how the infarct pattern and imaging characteristics can suggest an underlying cause.

Occlusion of a cervical or cerebral artery may cause acute ischemic stroke (AIS). Recent advances in AIS treatment by endovascular thrombectomy have led to more widespread use of advanced computed tomography (CT) imaging, including perfusion CT (PCT). This article reviews PCT for the evaluation of AIS patients.

Various imaging techniques play a role in the diagnosis of CNS vasculopathies, which comprise a heterogeneous group of disorders, including various noninflammatory and inflammatory etiologies. Noninflammatory vasculopathies include entities such as CADASIL, Susac, moyamoya, fibromuscular dysplasia, vasculopathy of connective tissue disorders, and reversible vasoconstriction syndrome. Inflammatory vasculopathies include vasculitides of different vessel sizes, primary angiitis of the CNS, vasculitis of systemic disease, and vasculitis secondary to specific causes. Miscellaneous etiology includes cerebral amyloid angiopathy, which has noninflammatory and inflammatory subtypes. This article discusses important clinical and imaging findings used to distinguish these disorders.

unique insight into preoperative planning for central nervous system (CNS) neoplasms by identifying areas of the brain effected or spared by the neoplasm. BOLD (blood-oxygen-level–dependent) fMR imaging can be reliably used to map eloquent cortex presurgically and is sufficiently accurate for neurosurgical planning. In patients with brain tumors undergoing neurosurgical intervention, fMR imaging can decrease postoperative morbidity. This article discusses the applications, significance, and interpretation of BOLD fMR imaging, and its applications in presurgical planning for CNS neoplasms.

Radiographic monitoring of posttreatment glioblastoma is important for clinical trials and determining next steps in management. Evaluation for tumor progression is confounded by the presence of treatment-related radiographic changes, making a definitive determination less straight-forward. The purpose of this article was to describe imaging tools available for assessing treatment response in glioblastoma, as well as to highlight the definitions, pathophysiology, and imaging features typical of true progression, pseudoprogression, pseudoresponse, and radiation necrosis.

Immunodeficiency can affect different components of the immune system and predispose to different types of opportunistic infections. For example, a defect in neutrophil or humoral immunity increases risk from disseminated infection by extracellular pathogens, whereas a defect in cytotoxic activity by natural killer cells or $CD8^+$ T lymphocytes increases risk from intracellular pathogens. The latter also increases risk from malignancies, due to impairment of normal immunosurveillance against abnormal neoplastic cells. The purpose of this article is to discuss central nervous system lesions that may be seen in the immunocompromised patient, organized into 5 categories: bacterial, fungal, parasitic, viral, and neoplastic.

PROGRAM OBJECTIVE

The objective of the *Radiologic Clinics of North America* is to keep practicing radiologists and radiology residents up to date with current clinical practice in radiology by providing timely articles reviewing the state of the art in patient care.

TARGET AUDIENCE

Practicing radiologists, radiology residents, and other healthcare professionals who provide patient care utilizing radiologic findings.

LEARNING OBJECTIVES

Upon completion of this activity, participants will be able to:

1. Review the role of MR perfusion and spectroscopy in the management of and treatment plans for brain neoplasms
2. Discuss the current state of imaging for acute ischemic stroke.
3. Recognize relevant clinical, molecular, and imaging features that are unique to pediatric brain tumors.

ACCREDITATION

The Elsevier Office of Continuing Medical Education (EOCME) is accredited by the Accreditation Council for Continuing Medical Education (ACCME) to provide continuing medical education for physicians.

The EOCME designates this journal-based CME activity for a maximum of 11 *AMA PRA Category 1 Credit*(s)™. Physicians should claim only the credit commensurate with the extent of their participation in the activity.

All other healthcare professionals requesting continuing education credit for this enduring material will be issued a certificate of participation.

DISCLOSURE OF CONFLICTS OF INTEREST

The EOCME assesses conflict of interest with its instructors, faculty, planners, and other individuals who are in a position to control the content of CME activities. All relevant conflicts of interest that are identified are thoroughly vetted by EOCME for fair balance, scientific objectivity, and patient care recommendations. EOCME is committed to providing its learners with CME activities that promote improvements or quality in healthcare and not a specific proprietary business or a commercial interest.

The planning committee, staff, authors and editors listed below have identified no financial relationships or relationships to products or devices they or their spouse/life partner have with commercial interest related to the content of this CME activity:

Behnam Badie, MD; Jacqueline Bello, MD; Judah Burns, MD; Ammar A. Chaudhry, MD; Abbas Chaudhry, PhD; Mike Chen, MD, PhD; Melissa M. Chen, MD; Gloria C. Chiang, MD; Edward J. Ebani, MD; Karem Gharzeddine, MD; Maryam Gul, MD; Ajay Gupta, MD, MS; Vaios Hatzoglou, MD; Steven Hetts, MD; Andrei I. Holodny, MD, PhD (hon), FACR; Camilo Jaimes, MD; Rahul Jandial, MD, PhD; Alison Kemp; Rajkamal Khangura, MD; Ashley Knight-Greenfield, MD; Kelly K. Koeller, MD; Pradeep Kuttysankaran; Alex Levitt, MD; Christie M. Malayil Lincoln, MD; Alicia Meng, MD; Frank Miller; Sohaib Naim, BSc; Joel Jose Quitlong Nario, BS; Tina Young Poussaint, MD, FACR; Javier M. Romero, MD; Pamela W. Schaefer, MD; Robert Y. Shih, MD; Shira E. Slasky, MD; Jae W. Song, MD; Jennifer E. Soun, MD; Sara B. Strauss, MD; Eric S. Sussman, MD; John Vassallo; Kevin Yuqi Wang, MD; Max Wintermark, MD; Richard Zampolin, MD.

The planning committee, staff, authors and editors listed below have identified financial relationships or relationships to products or devices they or their spouse/life partner have with commercial interest related to the content of this CME activity:

Jeremy J. Heit, MD, PhD: is a consultant/advisor for Medtronic and MicroVention, Inc.

Robert J. Young, MD: has received research support from NordicNeuroLab, Agios, Inc., Puma Biotechnology, Inc., and ICON plc.

UNAPPROVED/OFF-LABEL USE DISCLOSURE

The EOCME requires CME faculty to disclose to the participants:

1. When products or procedures being discussed are off-label, unlabelled, experimental, and/or investigational (not US Food and Drug Administration [FDA] approved); and
2. Any limitations on the information presented, such as data that are preliminary or that represent ongoing research, interim analyses, and/or unsupported opinions. Faculty may discuss information about pharmaceutical agents that is outside of FDA-approved labelling. This information is intended solely for CME and is not intended to promote off-label use of these medications. If you have any questions, contact the medical affairs department of the manufacturer for the most recent pre-scribing information.

TO ENROLL

To enroll in the *Radiologic Clinics of North America* Continuing Medical Education program, call customer service at 1-800-654-2452 or sign up online at http://www.theclinics.com/home/cme. The CME program is available to subscribers for an additional annual fee of USD 327.60.

METHOD OF PARTICIPATION

In order to claim credit, participants must complete the following:

1. Complete enrolment as indicated above.
2. Read the activity.
3. Complete the CME Test and Evaluation. Participants must achieve a score of 70% on the test. All CME Tests and Evaluations must be completed online.

CME INQUIRIES/SPECIAL NEEDS

For all CME inquiries or special needs, please contact elsevierCME@elsevier.com.

RADIOLOGIC CLINICS OF NORTH AMERICA

THE CLINICS ARE AVAILABLE ONLINE!
Access your subscription at:
www.theclinics.com

Preface
Updates in Brain Imaging

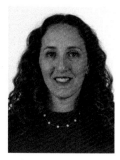

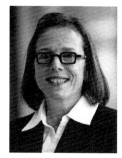

Shira E. Slasky, MD   Jacqueline A. Bello, MD, FACR
Editors

Neuroradiology has seen many advances in the past few years, placing the radiologist in a crucial role. Large trials have demonstrated the efficacy of thrombectomy for large vessel occlusions in stroke, emphasizing the importance of triaging patients for intervention. Genomics has become central to the classification of brain neoplasms, culminating in the 2016 World Health Organization classification of brain tumors. Advanced imaging techniques, such as functional MR imaging, diffusion tensor imaging, perfusion, and MR spectroscopy, have added value in tumor diagnosis, surgical planning, and surveillance. This *Radiologic Clinics of North America* issue aims to revisit many commonly encountered entities, viewing them through the lens of recent updates.

While the issue provides a general overview of stroke imaging along with an in-depth review of stroke causes and their typical imaging patterns, it also reviews computed tomographic perfusion and how it is used to triage patients for management of acute stoke. One article thoroughly addresses central nervous system (CNS) vasculopathies, organizing them based on the latest classification system. Another article takes an in-depth look at posterior reversible encephalopathy syndrome and reversible cerebral vasoconstriction syndrome, including pertinent pathophysiology, and clinical and imaging findings. An updated classification of brain tumors is reviewed, with emphasis on the importance of genetic markers and prognostic stratification through imaging. Another section focuses on imaging of glioblastoma after treatment.

The final topic presents a thorough review of CNS lesions in immunocompromised patients. These articles provide excellent coverage of many of the latest advances in neuroradiology.

We thank each of the authors for their dedication and effort in preparing this issue of *Radiologic Clinics of North America*. The contributors are experts in the field of neuroradiology and represent various institutions, bringing diverse cases to this issue. Their exceptional work products provide an in-depth review of many of the latest advances in brain imaging, which we are delighted to share with you.

Shira E. Slasky, MD
Division of Neuroradiology
Department of Radiology
Albert Einstein College of Medicine
Montefiore Medical Center
111 East 210 Street
Bronx, NY 10467-2490, USA

Jacqueline A. Bello, MD, FACR
Division of Neuroradiology
Department of Radiology
Albert Einstein College of Medicine
Montefiore Medical Center
111 East 210 Street
Bronx, NY 10467-2490, USA

E-mail addresses:
sslasky@montefiore.org (S.E. Slasky)
jbello@montefiore.org (J.A. Bello)

Radiol Clin N Am 57 (2019) xiii
https://doi.org/10.1016/j.rcl.2019.07.010
0033-8389/19/© 2019 Published by Elsevier Inc.

Imaging of Acute Stroke
Current State

Steven Hetts, MD[a], Rajkamal Khangura, MD[b],*

KEYWORDS

- Acute ischemic stroke • Endovascular therapy • Thrombectomy • Computer tomography perfusion
- Neurointervention • Large-vessel occlusion

KEY POINTS

- Endovascular therapy for large-vessel occlusions may now be performed up to 24 hours after time last known well.
- Stroke systems of care should be protocolized to allow for rapid, efficient stroke imaging to allow for faster revascularization.
- Efficient, rapid neuroimaging differentiates acute ischemic stroke from stroke mimics, identifies intracranial and extracranial occlusions, and delineates cranio-cervical vascular anatomy, extent of core infarction, volume of salvageable brain (ischemic penumbra), and status of leptomeningeal collaterals.

INTRODUCTION

Acute ischemic stroke (AIS) affects up to 1 in 6 adults in their lifetime and is the leading cause of long-term severe disability in North America, with nearly 800,000 cases of AIS in the United States annually. Ischemic stroke represents most acute stroke events (87%), whereas hemorrhagic stroke represents a minority of cases (13%).[1] Approximately 30% of ischemic strokes involve acute large-vessel occlusion (LVO) of the intracranial arteries, predominantly involving the anterior circulation (internal carotid artery, middle cerebral artery, or anterior cerebral artery).[2] Overwhelmingly positive results from 5 randomized controlled trials published in 2015 supported the use of endovascular therapy (EVT) in LVO within the first 6 to 8 hours of stroke onset. More recent trials using advanced imaging to select patients with salvageable brain tissue have extended the LVO treatment window to 18 to 24 hours.[3,4] Meta-analysis of the major trials, the HERMES collaboration, confirmed

treatment benefit in nearly all subgroups and identified time to treatment as the primary predictor of good outcome (modified Rankin Scale score <2).[5] Diagnostic neuroimaging is essential in triaging stroke patients for intravenous thrombolysis therapy inclusion and, if LVO is identified, proceeding to endovascular therapy. Efficient, rapid neuroimaging differentiates AIS from stroke mimics, identifies intracranial and extracranial occlusions, delineates cranio-cervical vascular anatomy, extent of core infarction, volume of salvageable brain (ischemic penumbra), and status of leptomeningeal collaterals. This article discusses the current state of acute stroke imaging, focusing on imaging findings that have an impact on endovascular stroke treatment.

SYSTEMS OF STROKE CARE

The mantra "time is brain" encapsulates the goal of stroke intervention systems of care—streamlined diagnosis and rapid revascularization. Faster

No disclosures.
[a] Division of Neurointerventional Radiology, University of California, San Francisco, 505 Parnassus Avenue # M-380, San Francisco, CA 94143, USA; [b] Department of Radiology and Biomedical Imaging, Division of Neurointerventional Radiology, University of California, San Francisco, 505 Parnassus Avenue # M-380, San Francisco, CA 94143, USA
* Corresponding author.
E-mail address: rajkamal.khangura@ucsf.edu

radiologic.theclinics.com

diagnosis and recanalization of LVOs are associated with greater likelihood of a disability-free outcome. Clinical suspicion of AIS, activated in the field or the hospital, results in a cascade of events often with imaging as the rate-limiting step. Once prehospital or in-hospital stroke activation occurs, providers and staff involved in stroke treatment should also be notified; this includes the neuroradiologist. Initial noncontrast computed tomography (CT) interpretation, either at the scanner or in the reading room, begins the treatment algorithm for intravenous thrombolytic therapy and subsequent endovascular therapy. After noncontrast head CT, computed tomography angiography (CTA) covering from the left atrial appendage through the cranial vertex should be obtained. If the patient is beyond 6 hours from time last seen normal, then computed tomography perfusion (CTP) should be performed to determine extended window eligibility. Initial imaging should be protocolized to prevent delays associated with imaging. Protocolized imaging provides the greatest capture of patients presenting with LVOs. Additional components of a stroke protocol CT should include pre-set slice thickness, multiplanar reformats, and true axial images.

CT with CTA remains the clinical standard to evaluate for LVO because it was the primary noninvasive vascular imaging in the major trials, although some sites used MR imaging and magnetic resonance angiography (MRA) with similar results and speed. According to the 2018 American Heart Association guidelines, the data to support the routine use of MR imaging for in-window thrombectomy candidates are inadequate, and CT is preferred. In select patients who present in the extended time window, diffusion-weighted MR imaging provides definitive evaluation of the core infarct volume and perfusion MR imaging characterizes tissue mismatch/tissue at risk.[6] Use of MR imaging with MRA in this scenario must be balanced with rapid imaging acquisition and diagnosis to include patients for endovascular treatment.

In efforts to dramatically lower "door to tissue plasminogen activator" time and treat a greater percentage of patients with early thrombolysis, mobile stroke units have been developed; these are modified ambulances with an on-board CT scanner, technologist, critical care nurse, emergency medical service provider/paramedic, and neurologist. Patients are scanned using the mobile CT scanner to evaluate for exclusionary criteria for thrombolysis.

Lastly, direct transfer to the angiography suite is being evaluated, bypassing the emergency room and CT scanner to reduce "door-to-puncture" time. In this scenario, a CT and potentially CTA/CTP are acquired using cone-bean CT technology within the angiography suite. A pilot study in Barcelona demonstrated the feasibility and significant time reduction using this strategy in patients with high prehospital stroke scale scores.[7]

NEUROIMAGING
Noncontrast Head Computed Tomography

AIS remains a clinical diagnosis although treatment is centered around exclusionary criteria obtained from patient history and diagnostic imaging. CT imaging is the cornerstone of routine ischemic stroke imaging, followed by CTA and advanced imaging such as CTP or multiphase CTA in patients who present during the extended treatment window. The noncontrast head CT should be obtained from the vertex through C2, provided in true axial reconstructions and best viewed in 35-45/35-45 window/level settings. The primary objective of the head CT is to exclude patients from intravenous (IV) thrombolysis; these exclusionary criteria include evidence of hemorrhage, mass, and completed large infarction. In the absence of these findings, the patient remains a candidate for IV thrombolysis within the appropriate treatment time (currently within 4.5 hours after time last seen well in most centers). Additional findings suggestive of acute ischemia, although specific, are not sensitive. These include the hyperdense vessel sign, loss of insular ribbon sign, territorial gray-white differentiation loss, and rarely, sulcal effacement (seen toward the end of the acute ischemic phase and more commonly as a subacute ischemic finding).

Major findings that should be evaluated include

1. Evidence of hemorrhage, mass or mass effect, and hydrocephalus
2. Evidence of gray-white differentiation loss and assessment of Alberta Stroke Program Early Computed Tomography Score (ASPECTS) to characterize core infarction
3. Hyperdense vessel sign

Following the exclusion of stroke mimics and hemorrhage, the scan should be assessed for evidence of core infarction, best assessed with ASPECTS. The total volume of the middle cerebral artery territory is roughly 300 cm^3, divided into 10 anatomic regions, with each area representing approximately 30 cm^3 of brain tissue (**Fig. 1**). All slices from the lower ganglionic level through the cephalad aspect of the supraganglionic level should be assessed. Each area of hypoattenuation/ischemic change/core infarction results in subtraction of 1 point for each involved region

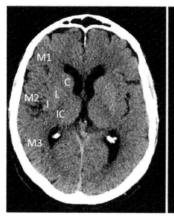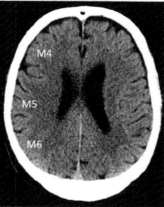

Fig. 1. Ten regions with 4 for ganglionic gray-matter structures: caudate (C); lentiform (L); internal capsule (IC); insular ribbon (I); and 6 for cortically based structures in the MCA territory: M1–M6.[8] (*From* Schröder, J., & Thomalla, G. (2017). A Critical Review of Alberta Stroke Program Early CT Score for Evaluation of Acute Stroke Imaging . *Frontiers in Neurology* . Retrieved from https://www.frontiersin.org/article/10.3389/fneur.2016.0024; with permission.)

from a normal score of 10. Level 1 evidence supports treatment of patients with ASPECTS greater than 6.

The dense vessel sign is suggestive of higher red blood cell (RBC) content within thrombus,[9] which seems to be secondary to a cardioembolic source of embolism (**Fig. 2**). Less dense thrombi may be suggestive of fibrin-rich, platelet-rich emboli, which typically arise from large-vessel atherosclerotic sources.[10] Lastly, a calcified embolus may be secondary to a chronically formed clot from a cardioembolic source or from an artery to artery embolus. Because these factors may affect the potential devices used during thrombectomy, this information should be promptly conveyed to the neurointerventionalist.

Patients who receive IV thrombolysis should then be evaluated with vessel imaging for evidence of

LVO, because this is amenable to EVT. Again, this imaging should be acquired immediately after the noncontrast CT head as part of the protocolized Stroke CT with CTA study.

Computed Tomography Angiography

A CTA of both the head and neck should then be performed, extending from the left atrial appendage through the vertex, and reconstructed in multiplanar reconstruction and maximum intensity projection (MIP) images for evaluation of the origin of the great vessels, carotid disease or narrowing, and the intracranial vasculature.[11] Given that time is of the essence, imaging is obtained without evaluating the patient's renal status.

Treatment planning should be considered when evaluating the CTA. Characterization of the aortic arch, patency of the independent origins of the great vessels as well as common origins should be reported (**Fig. 3**). The course and tortuosity of vessels should be described. Evaluation of the distal common carotid artery (CCA), internal carotid artery (ICA) bulb and proximal ICA should be documented to establish the potential source of stroke. Most strokes are cardioembolic, followed by artery to artery emboli from the carotid artery.

Intracranially, the length of occlusion should be described, because it may aid in device selection. In describing the middle cerebral artery (MCA) M1 segment, it should be noted that an early bifurcation of the MCA is considered an M1 location as long as it is within the horizontal segment of the sylvian fissure. Thrombus involving the bifurcation may involve the superior or inferior truck, representing M2 occlusions.

Occlusions are best seen on MIP slab images, and reconstructions should always be provided as part of the standard stroke protocol.

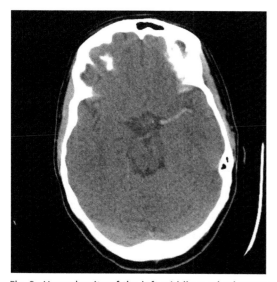

Fig. 2. Hyperdensity of the left middle cerebral artery M1 segment.

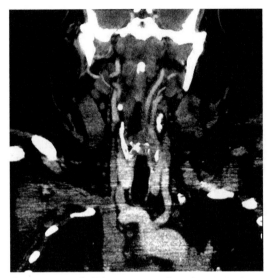

Fig. 3. Coronal CTA reconstruction demonstrates a common origin of the innominate artery and left common carotid artery.

Extending the Treatment Window for Patients with Large-Vessel Occlusion

Analysis of the 5 major trials revealed that patients can be stratified into 2 categories: patients with rapid expansion of the ischemic core (so-called fast progressors) and patients with slow growth of their ischemic core (so-called slow progressors). Their outcome seems to be determined primarily by their collaterals (**Fig. 4**).[12]

Two recent studies evaluating the role of thrombectomy in patients beyond the 6 hour time window demonstrated unequivocal benefit of mechanical thrombectomy between 6 and 16 hours (DEFUSE 3) and up to 24 hours (DAWN).[3,4] The principle behind these study populations was that, based on the HERMES pooled patient analysis, a subset of patients benefit from treatment in the extended window time period. This ability to maintain a small core volume despite late presentation is most likely explained by robust leptomeningeal collaterals.

Advanced imaging combined with automated processing may alert physicians to patients with undiagnosed LVO in the early window. Systems should be streamlined to reduce time to allow for rapid detection, diagnosis, thrombolysis, and transfer if LVO present. Protocolized studies for CTP in the extended window should be initiated according to the particular institution's policy, either up to 16 hours (DEFUSE 3) or up to 24 hours (DAWN).

Multiphase acquisition of head CTA to characterize leptomeningeal collaterals has been developed and pioneered by the Calgary/Alberta group (ESCAPE Trial).[13] Patients are characterized as having poor, intermediate, or robust collaterals, which can aid patient selection for the extended window patient.

Perfusion imaging is intended to identify patients with salvageable brain tissue (ischemic penumbra). The inclusion criteria of the 2 randomized control trials, DEFUSE 3 and DAWN, evaluating endovascular stroke treatment in the extended window are shown in **Table 1.**

Briefly, CTP is a time-resolved multiphase acquisition following a contrast bolus injection. Reconstructed images are then post processed to generate color maps of the mean transit time (MTT), time to peak (TTP), cerebral blood flow (CBF), and cerebral blood volume (CBV) parameters. The best estimation of the infarct core is an area of tissue with approximately 30% CBF

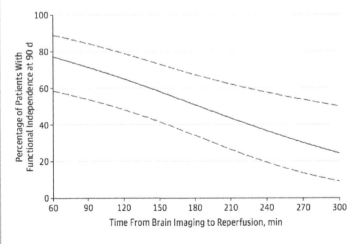

Fig. 4. The dashed lines reflect the 95% confidence interval range as well as reflecting patients with robust collaterals (*upper dashed line*) or low collaterals (*lower dashed line*), supporting both fast treatment and EVT for extended window patients with good collaterals and low core infarction. (*From* Saver JL, Goyal M, van der Lugt A, et al. Time to treatment with endovascular thrombectomy and outcomes from ischemic stroke: a meta-analysis endovascular thrombectomy and outcomes in ischemic stroke endovascular thrombectomy and outcomes in ischemic stroke. JAMA 2016;316(12):1279-89; with permission.)

Table 1
The inclusion criteria of the 2 randomized control trials, DEFUSE 3 and DAWN

	DEFUSE 3	DAWN
Age and baseline mRS	Age: 18–90 years Baseline mRS: 0–1	Age: At least 18 years Baseline mRS: 0–1
IV thrombolysis	tPA if started within 4.5 h of onset	tPA given with persistence of LVO or outside of tPA window
Time since last known well	6–16 h	6–24 h
Imaging	ASPECTS ≥6	No intracerebral hemorrhage on CT or MR imaging No evidence of stroke in >1/3 of MCA territory
Mismatch inclusion criteria	Initial core infarct volume <70 cm³ NIHSS ≥6 Ratio of volume of ischemic tissue to initial infarct volume of 1.8 or more Absolute volume of penumbra tissue of 15 cm³ or more (defined as Tmax >6 s using RAPID software)	Group A: >80 years NIHSS ≥ 10, core infarct <21 cm³ Group B: <80 year, NIHSS ≥10, core infarct <31 cm³ Group C: <80 years, NIHSS ≥20, core infarct 31–50 cm³
Occlusion location	ICA, MCA, or both	ICA, MCA, or both

Abbreviations: ICA, intracerebral hemorrhage; mRS, modified Rankin Scale; NIHSS, National Institutes of Health Stroke Scale.

compared with normal brain tissue.[14] Tissue at risk or ischemic penumbra is characterized by prolongation of MTT or delayed TTP/Tmax. The mismatch between areas of deceased CBF or CBV compared with prolongation of a time parameter reflects salvageable brain tissue (**Fig. 5**). This assessment forms the basis of treatment of patients in the extended treatment window.

PEARLS, PITFALLS, VARIANTS
Intracranial Atherosclerotic Disease

Acute plaque rupture of intracranial atherosclerosis may present similar to cardioembolic or artery to artery embolic stroke but typically does not respond to mechanical thrombectomy or thromboaspiration.[15] Treatment with a stentriever results in further platelet aggregation of the

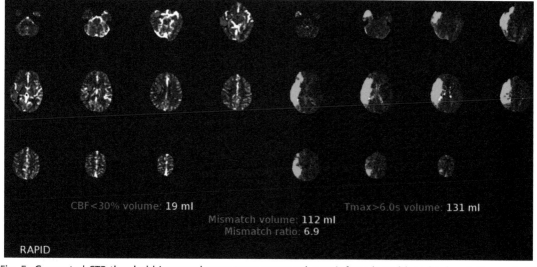

CBF<30% volume: **19 ml**   Tmax>6.0s volume: **131 ml**
Mismatch volume: **112 ml**
Mismatch ratio: **6.9**

RAPID

Fig. 5. Generated CTP threshold images demonstrate suspected core infarct (*purple*) and ischemic tissue at risk (*green*), representing a favorable mismatch profile. (*Courtesy of* Ischemaview RAPID.)

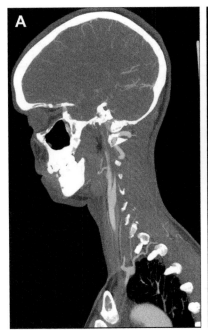
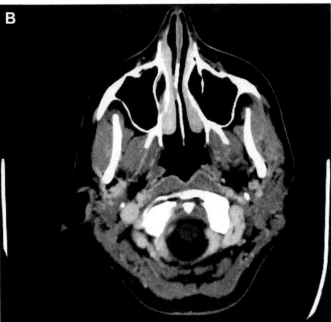

Fig. 6. (*A*) Sagittal CTA of the neck shows decreased opacification with tapered appearance of the proximal left ICA. (*B*) Post-contrast axial CT of the head in the same patient reveals a patent distal left cervical ICA, suggesting the initial nonopacification of the left cervical ICA represented a "pseudo-occlusion."

thrombus, and patients may ultimately require intravenous antiplatelet treatment, balloon angioplasty, or intracranial stenting. The noncontrast CT may suggest intracranial atherosclerotic disease (ICAD) with evidence of calcium deposition in the vessel wall or absence of a hyperdense vessel sign. Common locations of intracranial atherothrombotic occlusions are in the mid to distal MCAs and mid basilar artery.[16] Evidence of other sites of intracranial atherosclerosis (excluding the carotid siphons) may suggest ICAD. CTP and multiphase CTA may reveal well-developed collaterals and a favorable mismatch profile, likely reflective of the chronicity of the underlying lesion.

Chronic Extracranial Occlusion/Near-Total Occlusion

Chronic occlusions of the extracranial circulation pose clinical challenges, because there is no intracranial LVO but upstream narrowing or occlusion with greater stress placed on the circle of Willis or leptomeningeal collaterals. In general, recent extracranial carotid occlusions are not typically treated, although revascularization may be appropriate in certain clinical scenarios (increasing NIHSS, recurrent strokes). Symptomatic ICA occlusion requires revascularization within 14 days of the stroke.[17] The degree of stenosis, the location relative to both the mandible and

cervical vertebral level, tortuosity of the vessel, length of stenosis, and degree of peripheral calcification should be reported to help determine eligibility for carotid endarterectomy versus carotid stenting.

Tandem Occlusions

Tandem occlusions consist of concomitant intracranial LVO and ipsilateral extracranial ICA occlusion, occurring in approximately 10% to 20% of cases of AIS.[18] Treatment is often complex, influenced by the ability to cross the proximal occlusion, the volume of the core infarction, the degree of success of intracranial revascularization, adequacy of circle of Willis collaterals, and extracranial lesion morphology. Common causes of tandem occlusion include acute occlusion of a previously nearly occluded common/internal carotid artery, acute plaque rupture of an ICA atherosclerotic lesion with distal embolization, or carotid dissection with thrombus formation and embolization. First-pass CTA limits the evaluation of a tandem lesion, but delayed imaging may help evaluate vascular patency, vessel contour, distal collapse of the ICA, string sign, or filling defect suggestive of an ulcerated plaque. During the arterial phase of acquisition, there may be absence of opacification of the distal CCA or proximal ICA. This is typically explained by 2 potential processes: "pseudo-occlusion" or tandem occlusion.

Pseudo-occlusions of the cervical carotid occur with occlusion of the ICA terminus or in an isolated hemisphere with MCA M1 occlusion (**Fig. 6**). Poor vascular opacification of the cervical ICA occurs because there are no branches of the cervical ICA; therefore poor antegrade flow results in poor/incomplete opacification during the arterial phase of imaging.

A post-contrast scan may be obtained to evaluate for delayed filling of the extracranial vasculature, which may appear to be occluded, hence the so-called pseudo-occlusion on the first-pass angiographic phase of imaging.

Malignant Pattern of Collaterals

Patients with poor collaterals have poor opacification of vessels in the occluded territory, which is associated with more rapid core infarction expansion and poorer prognosis (**Fig. 7**).[19] Typically, some degree of arterial and venous filling is seen as a result of collateral arterial filling from anterior cerebral artery–MCA or posterior cerebral artery–MCA leptomeningeal collaterals. Patients with a so-called malignant pattern of collaterals will have a rapidly expanding infarct core unless the LVO is opened. For these patients, time is of the utmost importance. This should be promptly recognized and relayed to the neurointerventionalist.

Basilar Artery Occlusions

Posterior circulation LVOs, specifically basilar artery occlusions, were not included in the major randomized studies. To date, there are no randomized studies evaluating modern era endovascular therapy devices for treatment of basilar occlusions. Retrospective data suggest that endovascular therapy is safe and effective for basilar occlusions.[20] Occlusion of the proximal and middle segments of the basilar artery are more likely to reflect underlying ICAD.[21] Distal occlusions and evidence of thalamic infarctions are more often seen with embolic stroke. Guideline recommendations from the Society of Neurointerventional Surgery recommend imaging evaluation initially with CT/CTA with possible diffusion-weighted imaging for late arrivals, as institutionally defined, to exclude those with a poor pc-ASPECTS (posterior circulation ASPECTS) or large core infarction.[22]

WHAT THE REFERRING PHYSICIAN NEEDS TO KNOW

Noncontrast CT imaging should provide exclusionary reasons why patients are not candidates

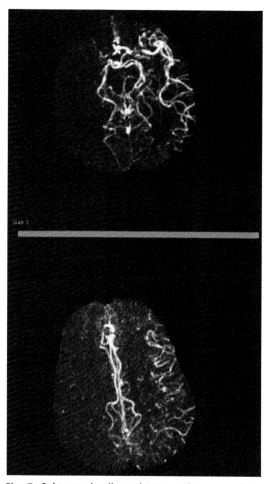

Fig. 7. Subtracted collapsed MIP axial images of the circle of Willis reveal a right ICA terminus occlusion with little contrast opacification of the right MCA territory, suggestive of poor collaterals, a malignant collateral pattern. (*Courtesy of* Ischemaview RAPID.)

for thrombolysis, such as hemorrhage, mass, or hydrocephalus. In the absence of these exclusionary imaging findings and other patient factors determined by their medical history, intravenous thrombolysis can be administered.

A dense vessel sign is highly specific for LVO, specifically, an RBC-rich thrombus. Measurement of the thrombus length provides some clinical value to size the stentriever or rule out primary aspiration (which is less favorable for longer thrombi). Ischemic change should be reported as part of the patient's ASPECTS, which can be reported as a range (eg, ASPECTS of approximately 8–10). CTA establishes the LVO and in the absence of extensive early ischemic change (ASPECTS <6), patients are candidates for EVT. Neurointerventionalists benefit from learning about aortic arch anat6omic variants, cervical carotid disease status, and vascular tortuosity. Tandem lesions secondary to carotid artery atherosclerosis or ICA dissection present a dilemma for the neurointerventionalists; earlier diagnosis provides the opportunity to plan intervention. CTP/multiphase CTA best evaluates the ischemic tissue at risk and potential collaterals, respectively. CBV and MTT/TTP should be reported along with parameter ratios. The quality of collaterals should be reported in the impression. If present, malignant-type collaterals should be reported immediately to the neuerointerventionalist.

SUMMARY

Recent randomized control trials demonstrate the benefit of thrombectomy potentially up to 24 hours in selected patients. CT remains the standard and primary mode of imaging for acute stroke. Treatment benefit is seen in the absence of extensive early ischemic change. Diagnostic imaging plays a central role in providing efficient exclusionary criteria for thrombolysis, diagnosis of LVO, and selecting appropriate patients in the extended window based on expedient automated advanced imaging software. Radiologists may aid neurointerventionalists with the diagnosis of LVO on the noncontrast head CT, potentially bypassing noninvasive vascular imaging. In addition, identification of potential ICAD or tandem lesions may change the course of treatment, benefiting the patient's outcome.

ACKNOWLEDGMENTS

Dr Steven Hetts acknowledges NIH grant R01EB012031 as a source of funding.

REFERENCES

1. Benjamin EJ, Blaha MJ, Chiuve SE, et al, on behalf of the American Heart Association Statistics Committee and Stroke Statistics Subcommittee. Heart disease and stroke statistics—2017 update: a report from the American Heart Association. Circulation 2017;135:e229–445.
2. Go S. Posterior circulation ischemic stroke. Mo Med 2015;112(3):192–6.
3. Albers GW, Marks MP, Kemp S, et al. Thrombectomy for stroke at 6 to 16 hours with selection by perfusion imaging. N Engl J Med 2018;378(8):708–18.
4. Nogueira RG, Jadhav AP, Haussen DC, et al. Thrombectomy 6 to 24 hours after stroke with a mismatch between deficit and infarct. N Engl J Med 2017; 378(1):11–21.
5. Goyal M, Menon BK, van Zwam WH, et al. Endovascular thrombectomy after large-vessel ischaemic stroke: a meta-analysis of individual patient data from five randomised trials. Lancet 2016; 387(10029):1723–31.
6. Powers WJ, Rabinstein AA, Ackerson T, et al. 2018 Guidelines for the early management of patients with acute ischemic stroke: a guideline for healthcare professionals from the American Heart Association/American Stroke Association. Stroke 2018; 49(3):e46–99.
7. Ribo M, Boned S, Rubiera M, et al. Direct transfer to angiosuite to reduce door-to-puncture time in thrombectomy for acute stroke. J Neurointerv Surg 2018; 10(3):221–4.
8. Schröder J, Thomalla G. A critical review of Alberta Stroke Program early CT score for evaluation of acute stroke imaging. Front Neurol 2017;7:245.
9. Liebeskind DS, Sanossian N, Yong WH, et al. CT and MRI early vessel signs reflect clot composition in acute stroke. Stroke 2011;42(5):1237–43.
10. Benson JC, Fitzgerald ST, Kadirvel R, et al. Clot permeability and histopathology: is a clot's perviousness on CT imaging correlated with its histologic composition? J Neurointerv Surg 2019. https://doi.org/10.1136/neurintsurg-2019-014979.
11. de Lucas EM, Sánchez E, Gutiérrez A, et al. CT protocol for acute stroke: tips and tricks for general radiologists. Radiographics 2008;28(6):1673–87.
12. Rocha M, Jovin TG. Fast versus slow progressors of infarct growth in large vessel occlusion stroke. Stroke 2017;48(9):2621–7.
13. Menon BK, d'Esterre CD, Qazi EM, et al. Multiphase CT angiography: a new tool for the imaging triage of patients with acute ischemic stroke. Radiology 2015; 275(2):510–20.
14. Campbell BC, Christensen S, Levi CR, et al. Cerebral blood flow is the optimal CT perfusion parameter for assessing infarct core. Stroke 2011;42(12):3435–40.
15. Jang-Hyun B, Moon KB, Hoe HJ, et al. Outcomes of endovascular treatment for acute intracranial atherosclerosis–related large vessel occlusion. Stroke 2018;49(11):2699–705.
16. Arenillas JF. Intracranial atherosclerosis. Stroke 2011;42(1_suppl_1):S20–3.
17. Sacco RL, Adams R, Albers G, et al. Guidelines for prevention of stroke in patients with ischemic stroke or transient ischemic attack. Stroke 2006;37(2): 577–617.
18. Marta R, Marc R, Raquel D-M, et al. Tandem internal carotid artery/middle cerebral artery occlusion. Stroke 2006;37(9):2301–5.
19. Souza LCS, Yoo AJ, Chaudhry ZA, et al. Malignant CTA collateral profile is highly specific for large admission DWI infarct core and poor outcome in acute stroke. AJNR Am J Neuroradiol 2012;33(7):1331–6.
20. Dong Hun K, Cheolkyu J, Woong Y, et al. Endovascular thrombectomy for acute basilar artery occlusion: a multicenter retrospective observational study. J Am Heart Assoc 2018;7(14):e009419.

21. Lee YY, Yoon W, Kim SK, et al. Acute basilar artery occlusion: differences in characteristics and outcomes after endovascular therapy between patients with and without underlying severe atherosclerotic stenosis. AJNR Am J Neuroradiol 2017;38(8): 1600–4.

22. Kayan Y, Meyers PM, Prestigiacomo CJ, et al. Current endovascular strategies for posterior circulation large vessel occlusion stroke: report of the Society of NeuroInterventional Surgery Standards and Guidelines Committee. J Neurointerv Surg 2019. https://doi.org/10.1136/neurintsurg-2019-014873.

Causes of Acute Stroke
A Patterned Approach

Ashley Knight-Greenfield, MD, Joel Jose Quitlong Nario, BS, Ajay Gupta, MD, MS*

KEYWORDS

- Stroke • Infarct • Ischemic • Hemorrhagic • Imaging • Cause

KEY POINTS

- Emergent imaging is performed on a high proportion of patients presenting with acute stroke symptoms; as such, imaging plays an important role in early diagnosis and management.
- Determining the cause of an acute stroke is critical for clinicians to initiate appropriate therapy.
- Imaging patterns of acute stroke can suggest the cause, and therefore aid in appropriate management.
- Once large vessel atherosclerosis, small vessel disease, and cardioembolic sources have been excluded, unusual causes should be considered.

INTRODUCTION

Acute stroke is a leading cause of morbidity and mortality in the United States and worldwide, with more than 750,000 cases and 140,000 deaths in the United States each year.[1,2] In the United States, patients who arrive at a hospital emergency department with acute stroke symptoms often undergo immediate computed tomography (CT) scanning, often before detailed clinical evaluation. Therefore, imaging has a critical role in early diagnosis of stroke. In addition to aiding in diagnosis of acute stroke, patterns of infarction on imaging can suggest a cause, which not only influences immediate management strategies, but also informs optimal secondary prevention therapies to prevent stroke recurrence. It is important to recognize these patterns to better guide image evaluation, recommend appropriate additional imaging as necessary, and ultimately arrive at the underlying cause. This article reviews imaging patterns and secondary findings that can assist in determining the cause of acute stroke.

ISCHEMIC STROKE

Ischemic strokes, which account for most infarcts, can be subdivided based on cause. The Trial of Org 10172 in Acute Stroke Treatment (TOAST) is a system developed to categorize subtypes of ischemic strokes and therefore guide proper management[3] (**Box 1**).

Large Artery Atherosclerosis

Infarctions larger than 15 to 20 mm, involving the cortex, cerebellum, brainstem, and subcortical regions, are usually caused by large vessel disease arising from atherosclerosis of cervical or proximal intracranial vessels,[3–5] comprising a major cause of acute stroke, ranging from 30% to 43%.[5] Evaluation of the cervical and intracranial vasculature is critical when large vessel atherosclerosis is suspected as the cause of acute infarction. The mechanism of infarction secondary to atherosclerosis of the extracranial vasculature is a combination of low-flow states and artery-to-artery emboli, with the latter thought to be the greater contributing factor.[6]

Disclosure: The authors have nothing to disclose.
Department of Radiology, Weill Cornell Medicine, 525 East 68th Street, New York, NY 10065, USA
* Corresponding author.
E-mail address: ajg9004@med.cornell.edu

Radiol Clin N Am 57 (2019) 1093–1108
https://doi.org/10.1016/j.rcl.2019.07.007

radiologic.theclinics.com

Box 1
Trial of Org 10172 in acute stroke treatment classification

- Large artery atherosclerosis (embolus or thrombosis)
- Cardioembolic
- Small vessel occlusion (lacune)
- Stroke of other determined cause, or unusual cause
- Stroke of undetermined cause
  - Two or more causes identified
  - Negative evaluation
  - Incomplete evaluation

The TOAST classification was developed to categorize causes of acute ischemic stroke. It is a useful way to categorize stroke in order to guide management decisions.

Anterior circulation infarcts from carotid atherosclerosis most commonly involve the middle cerebral artery (MCA),[5] resulting in a territorial infarction that involves the deep gray matter and cortex. Such infarcts typically involve the central portion of the brain, including the anterior parietal lobe, the posterior frontal lobe, and the superior temporal lobe (**Fig. 1**). The anterior cerebral artery (ACA) territory is frequently spared, because of an intact circle of Willis.[7] Proximal intracranial vascular disease is also under the purview of large artery atherosclerosis. Multiple mechanisms are postulated regarding the pathogenesis of stroke in these cases, including artery-to-artery emboli, in situ thromboembolism, and hemodynamic impairment[6] (**Fig. 2**).

Large vessel atherosclerosis affecting the vertebrobasilar system may also produce a specific set of imaging patterns. For example, in the setting of proximal or middle basilar artery occlusion, large

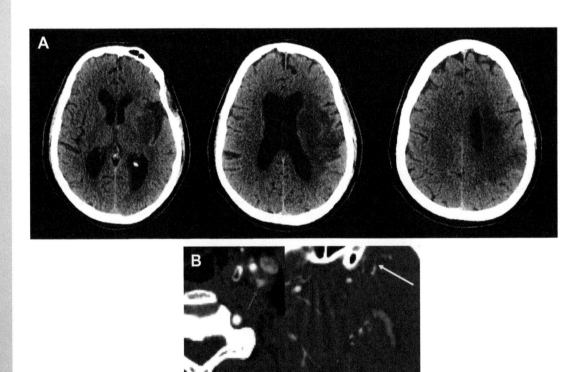

Fig. 1. A 54-year-old man presenting with altered mental status. (*A*) Axial CT images show an acute left MCA territory infarction involving the left insular cortex, basal ganglia, posterior frontal, and anterior parietal lobes. (*B*) Axial images from CT angiography (computed tomography) of the head and neck show moderate to severe stenosis of the proximal left ICA (*red arrow*) and left MCA thrombus involving the distal M1 and proximal M2 segments (*yellow arrow*).

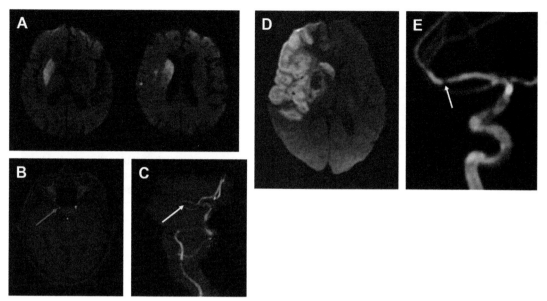

Fig. 2. Anterior circulation infarctions. (A) A 96-year-old woman with history of aortic valve repair on Coumadin presenting with acute-onset left hemiparesis. Axial diffusion-weighted magnetic resonance (MR) shows infarctions involving both deep gray matter and cortex, typical of an MCA territory infarction. (B) Axial MR angiography (magnetic resonance) time of flight (TOF) shows stenosis of the right intracranial ICA (*red arrow*). (C) Three-dimensional (3D) maximum intensity projection (MIP) image shows occlusion of the M1 segment of the right MCA (*yellow arrow*), with infarction probably secondary to a combination of hemodynamic impairment and artery-to-artery emboli. (D) A 73-year-old woman with hypertension and hyperlipidemia presenting with acute right MCA syndrome. Axial diffusion-weighted image shows infarct involving the right frontal lobe and basal ganglia in an MCA distribution. (E) 3D MIP from MRA head shows luminal narrowing of the right M1/M2 junction of the MCA (*white arrow*).

infarctions are usually seen in the pons as well as the cerebellum, bilateral inferomedial temporal lobes, occipital lobes, and posterior thalami (Fig. 3). Distal basilar occlusions usually involve the midbrain and thalami, and this is one of the few instances in which bilateral infarctions are seen in the setting of large vessel atherosclerosis.[8] Infarction of the lateral medulla should prompt radiologists to evaluate the distal vertebral artery, because this is often caused by occlusion of the posterior inferior cerebellar artery, clinically resulting in a lateral medullary syndrome.[9]

External border-zone infarcts are cortical infarcts that occur at the zones between the anterior, middle, and posterior cerebral artery (PCA) territories. Although the cause of these infarcts is not well understood, the prevailing theory is that they result from a combination of embolic phenomena and hypoperfusion.[10,11] Hypoperfusion may be secondary to actual hemodynamic compromise from stenosis, or caused by these areas being less well perfused at baseline. This condition, in turn, can lead to impaired washout in the setting of an embolic event.[10] In contrast, internal border-zone infarcts are more often caused by proximal stenoses or

hemodynamic compromise, because the lenticulostriate vessels supplying these regions have the lowest perfusion pressure (Fig. 4).[12] Posterior circulation border-zone infarcts are less common and, when unilateral, are more often caused by an embolic source from the anterior circulation in the setting of a fetal-type PCA[11,13] (Fig. 5).

When any of the imaging patterns discussed earlier are encountered, it is critical to evaluate the vasculature for large vessel atherosclerosis as the cause of acute stroke. Such evaluation may be performed with CT angiography (CTA), magnetic resonance (MR) angiography (MRA), or digital subtraction angiography (DSA). In addition, using MR imaging sequences beyond diffusion-weighted imaging may shed further light on infarct cause. For example, T2 fluid-attenuated inversion recovery (FLAIR) hyperintensity within intracranial vasculature may suggest slow flow caused by more proximal vascular disease (Fig. 6A). A serpiginous hypointense structure seen on susceptibility-weighted images may indicate thromboembolus in a distal vessel (Fig. 6B). A hyperdense MCA may be seen on initial noncontrast CT (Fig. 6C).

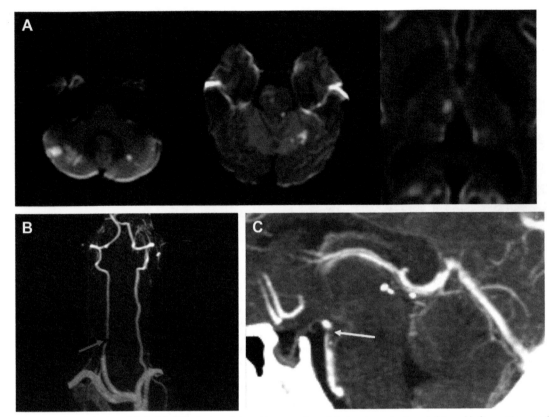

Fig. 3. Basilar occlusion. (*A*) Axial diffusion-weighted images show bilateral cerebellar, right and left pontine, and right thalamic infarcts. (*B*) 3D MIP image from MRA shows severe stenosis of the V1/V2 segment of the right vertebral artery (*red arrow*). (*C*) Sagittal MIP image from CTA head shows near-complete occlusion of the distal basilar artery (*yellow arrow*), which extended into the proximal PCAs.

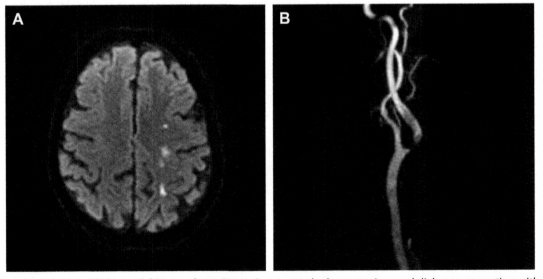

Fig. 4. A 72-year-old man with history of transient ischemic attacks, hypertension, and diabetes, presenting with right arm numbness. (*A*) Axial diffusion-weighted image shows acute infarction in an internal border zone distribution in the left frontoparietal lobes. (*B*) 3D MIP from MRA of the neck shows severe stenosis of the proximal cervical ICA.

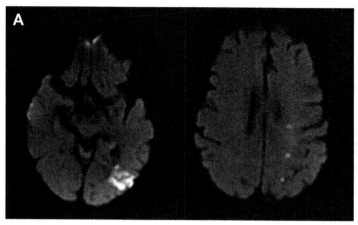
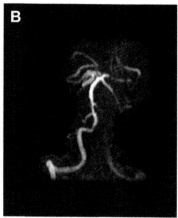

Fig. 5. A 75-year-old man with history of type 2 diabetes mellitus, hypercholesterolemia, hypertension, presenting with word-finding difficulty and right facial droop. (A) Axial diffusion-weighted images show acute infarctions involving MCA/PCA border-zone territories. (B) 3D MIP from MRA head shows complete lack of flow in the left V4 vertebral artery, as well as multifocal stenoses of the left PCA, both of which likely contributed to the border zone infarction.

Cardioembolic

Cardioembolic sources account for 20% to 31% of acute ischemic infarctions.[5,14] Such infarcts most often present on MR imaging as multiple foci of restricted diffusion involving multiple vascular territories, which are often bilateral[15] (Fig. 7). When this pattern is identified, it is critical to consider further evaluation of the heart, including additional diagnostic imaging. There are several causes of cardioembolic disease, including atrial fibrillation, myocardial infarction with left ventricular thrombus, and infective or inflammatory endocarditis. In addition, emboli may originate from aortic arch disorder, which can be missed on routine transthoracic echo; such cases can lead to bilateral infarctions as well.[16]

When isolated ACA infarctions are seen, a cardioembolic source should be considered, although there is debate as to the most common cause (Fig. 8A). Some studies have shown that the cause is more often cardioembolic,[17,18] whereas others have shown it is more often secondary to large vessel atherosclerosis of the ACA itself, the latter

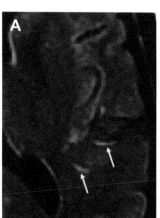
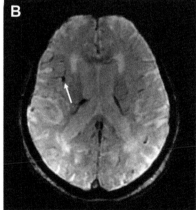
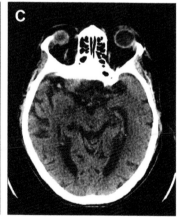

Fig. 6. (A) A 33-year-old woman presenting with confusion and aphasia, found to have a left MCA territory infarction and nonocclusive left M2 thrombus. Axial T2 FLAIR shows increased signal within multiple left MCA branches (yellow arrows) secondary to slow flow from the proximal partial occlusion. (B) A 94-year-old woman presenting with speech difficulties and left facial droop, found to have right MCA territory infarction. Susceptibility-weighted sequences show a tubular area of blooming in the anterior sylvian fissure, consistent with thromboembolus (white arrow). (C) A 90-year-old woman with history of congestive heart failure, hypertension, hyperlipidemia, presenting with left hemiparesis and dysarthria. Initial axial noncontrast head CT shows a dense right MCA (red arrow).

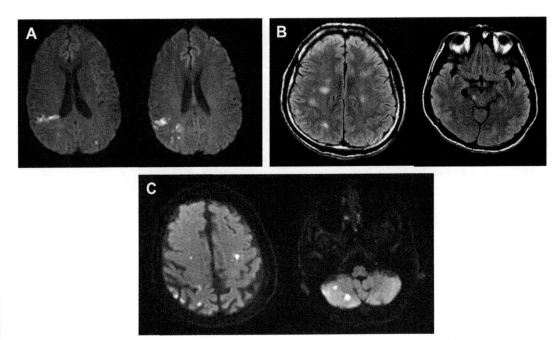

Fig. 7. Multiple bilateral infarctions from cardioembolic source. (A) Axial diffusion-weighted MR images in a 36-year-old woman with systemic lupus erythematous and Libman-Sacks endocarditis. (B) Axial T2 FLAIR images in a 38-year-old male intravenous drug abuser with bacterial endocarditis. (C) Axial diffusion-weighted MR images in a 79-year-old man with atrial fibrillation.

being more common in Asian populations.[19,20] Isolated ACA infarctions are less common than MCA infarctions.[5,7,17] When infarctions involve both the ACA and MCA territories, the cause is also often cardioembolic. For example, an acute myocardial infarction in a patient with atrial fibrillation may lead to distal emboli and decreased cardiac output[7] (Fig. 8B).

Small Artery Occlusion (Lacunar Infarction)

Small artery occlusions can be surmised as the cause of infarcts less than 20 mm, without evidence of other disorders, such as vascular disease, vasospasm, or a cardioembolic source.[4] These occlusions account for 10% to 23% of acute strokes.[5] Risk factors include diabetes and

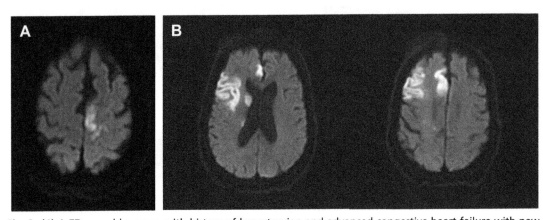

Fig. 8. (A) A 77-year-old woman with history of hypertension and advanced congestive heart failure with new-onset right hemiparesis. Axial diffusion-weighted MR image shows acute left ACA territory infarction likely secondary to cardioembolic source from advanced heart failure, because no vascular abnormality of the ACA was seen. (B) An 80-year-old man with history of prior stroke, atrial fibrillation, coronary artery disease, and hypertension presenting with new-onset left-sided weakness after collapse. Axial diffusion-weighted MR images reveal acute infarction in the right frontal cortex and right caudate head in a combined ACA/MCA distribution, likely cardioembolic in cause from known atrial fibrillation.

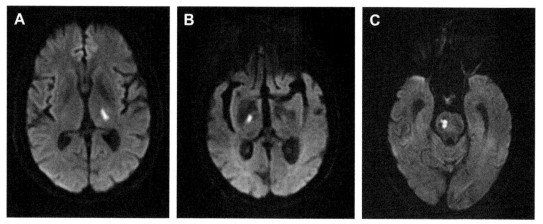

Fig. 9. Infarctions measuring less than 20 mm in the typical locations for small vessel infarctions, consistent with lacunar infarcts. (A) Axial diffusion-weighted MR shows acute infarct in the left thalamus in a hyperlipidemic smoker. (B) Axial diffusion-weighted MR shows acute infarct in the right internal capsule in a patient with multiple vascular risk factors. (C) Axial diffusion-weighted MR shows acute infarct in the right pons in a patient with hyperlipidemia and hypertension.

hypertension. Lacunar infarcts are seen most often in the basal ganglia, internal capsule, corona radiata, and brainstem (Fig. 9). PCA infarcts are more often lacunar in cause, and often present with typical clinical syndromes.[21] Exclusion of proximal vascular disease is critical to the diagnosis. Secondary findings on imaging that may suggest small vessel disease as the cause of infarction include presence of chronic lacunar infarcts, cerebral microbleeds, white matter ischemic disease, prominent perivascular spaces, and cerebral atrophy.[22]

Unusual Causes

Approximately 2% to 11% of ischemic strokes have unusual causes.[5,23] Although uncommon, it is important to consider atypical causes once common causes have been excluded, because this has important implications for management. Vasculopathies represent a large portion of unusual causes of stroke, in addition to other causes, such as hypercoagulable states, hematologic disorders, right-to-left vascular shunts, and arterial dissections. Although many of these disease processes look similar, certain patterns of vascular involvement and secondary findings on imaging may help elucidate the underlying cause.

Vasculopathies

Vasculopathies involving proximal vessels often result in territorial infarcts of perforating vessels supplying deep white matter and the basal ganglia. A component of subarachnoid hemorrhage may

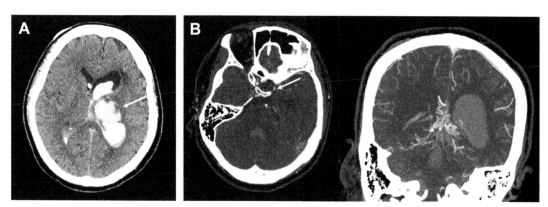

Fig. 10. A 49-year-old man with no known past medical history presented with acute-onset right-sided hemiparesis and confusion. (A) Axial noncontrast CT of the head shows a large left thalamic hematoma (arrow) with intraventricular extension. (B) Axial and MIP images from follow-up CTA show stenosis of the left cavernous ICA (arrow) as well as multiple collateral vessels, consistent with moyamoya.

also be seen.[24] Extensive collaterals are present in the setting of moyamoya and sickle cell disease. Moyamoya disease can present in both children and adults, usually as recurrent large territorial infarctions. In children, infarctions are often ischemic, whereas in adults they are more often hemorrhagic. Vascular imaging is critical and shows stenosis or occlusion of the distal internal carotid artery (ICA) and its proximal branches, with sparing of the posterior circulation.[7,25,26] The most salient imaging feature is the extensive collateral vascularity, best seen on vascular imaging (**Fig. 10**).

Basilar meningitis, as in the case of tuberculosis, can lead to arterial spasm and vasoconstriction of proximal vessels, resulting in infarction. Additional findings that may suggest this cause include involvement of the posterior circulation, unlike moyamoya, and involvement of perforating vessels, leading to basal ganglia and thalamic infarcts.[27] Secondary findings of communicating hydrocephalus, ventriculitis, and vasospasm further support this as a cause (**Fig. 11**). Acute septic meningitis from *Streptococcus pneumoniae*, *Neisseria meningitidis*, *Haemophilus influenzae*, and *Staphylococcus aureus* have been reported to cause infarction as well[28] (**Fig. 12**). Vasospasm may be seen on vascular imaging.[29]

Vasculopathies involving second-order and third-order arteries often result in cortical infarctions in distal vascular territories, typically without deep tissue involvement. These infarcts are also likely to be hemorrhagic. Contrast-enhanced MR angiography may show vessel wall enhancement. Causes include primary angiitis of the CNS (PACNS), granulomatosis with polyangiitis, polyarteritis nodosa, and sarcoid.[24] Infectious causes, such as syphilis and herpes zoster, may also affect second-order and third-order vessels. Herpes zoster occurs with reactivation of the latent virus, and is often indistinguishable from PACNS on imaging. It often presents with multiple infarcts, often involving the basal ganglia and subcortical white matter. Angiography may reveal segmental stenosis, thrombosis, and beading of the proximal MCA and ACA.[26] Subarachnoid hemorrhage may be seen[30,31] (**Fig. 13**).

Small vessel vasculopathies, such as Sjögren, collagen vascular disease, human immunodeficiency virus encephalitis, and radiation vasculopathy typically appear normal on angiography. Infarctions may be seen in deep gray structures, white matter, and subcortical regions. In contrast with multiple sclerosis, the white matter lesions seen with small vessel vasculopathy often

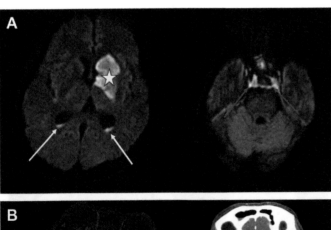

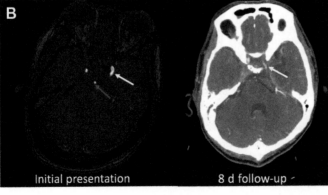

Fig. 11. A 55-year-old man with nasopharyngeal carcinoma presenting with altered mental status and fever, found to have *Streptococcus intermedius* meningitis. (*A*) Axial diffusion-weighted MR images show left basal ganglia and internal capsule infarction (*star*). On further inspection, the patient is noted to have mild ventriculomegaly and layering foci of restricted diffusion in the atria of the lateral ventricles, consistent with ventriculitis (*yellow arrows*). Restricted diffusion is also present in the basilar cisterns, consistent with basilar meningitis (*red arrows*). (*B*) Axial TOF image from MRA head at initial presentation and CTA head 8 days later. At 8-day follow-up, there is increased narrowing in the supraclinoid ICA (*yellow arrows*) and basilar artery (*red arrows*) secondary to vasospasm from basilar meningitis.

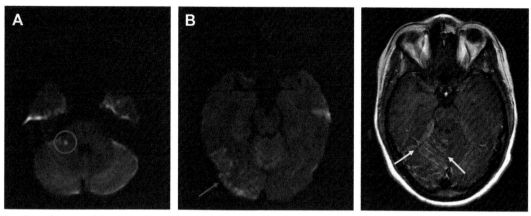

Fig. 12. A 27-year-old woman presenting with fever and acute visual loss after abscess drainage for lower extremity necrotizing fasciitis. (*A*) Axial diffusion-weighted MR image shows a small infarct in the right middle cerebellar peduncle (*circle*). (*B*) Secondary findings of sulcal restricted diffusion (*red arrow*) and leptomeningeal enhancement on axial T1 postcontrast MR (*yellow arrows*) suggest meningitis as the cause of infarction.

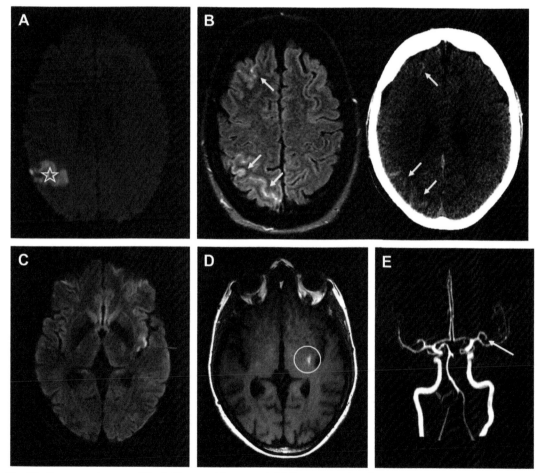

Fig. 13. Herpes zoster vasculitis. A 65-year-old woman initially presented with sudden-onset left hand weakness and facial droop. (*A*) Axial diffusion-weighted MR shows a right parietal infarct (*star*). (*B*) The patient was also noted to have failure of suppression of sulcal cerebrospinal fluid on T2 FLAIR, which corresponded to right convexity subarachnoid hemorrhage on noncontrast CT (*yellow arrows*). Vascular imaging was normal on initial presentation. (*C*) The patient returned 8 months later with right hand clumsiness and was found to have a new left insular infarct on axial diffusion-weighted MR (*red arrow*). (*D*) Axial T1-weighted image shows intrinsic T1 hyperintensity, consistent with hemorrhage (*circle*). (*E*) 3D MIP from MRA at that time reveals focal high-grade stenosis of an M2 branch of the left MCA (*yellow arrow*). Lumbar puncture revealed herpes zoster infection.

parallel the ventricles. These lesions often present at an earlier age and show rapid progression.[24]

Systemic lupus erythematous (SLE) is a collagen vascular disease that can result in small vessel vasculopathy (**Fig. 14**). Infarction pattern in lupus is nonspecific. More often than not, infarction is caused by secondary causes of the disease rather than vasculitis, such as cardiac valvular disease (Libman-Sacks endocarditis), hypercoagulability, atherosclerosis from hypertension and steroid treatment, and venous thrombosis. Secondary findings to look for include intracranial hemorrhage, and cerebral atrophy, with normal vascular imaging.[32]

Neoplastic vasculopathy is a result of vascular invasion secondary to neoplasm; affected patients may present with acute infarct. Vessel occlusion may be seen on angiography. Lymphoma is usually the cause, with the most common cause being non-Hodgkin. For example, diffuse large B-cell lymphoma (DLBCL) may present with acute infarcts and infarctlike lesions, which are diffusion restricting on MR imaging and show signal abnormality on T2-weighted sequences. Infarcts may involve the corpus callosum and periventricular white matter, and may be in a watershed distribution. In the case of DLBCL, small vessels are often involved, so angiography may be normal. Secondary findings include meningeal enhancement and central pontine hyperintensity, which may be secondary to venous congestion in the setting of vascular occlusion by tumor cells[33,34] (**Fig. 15**). Less common causes of neoplastic vasculopathy include

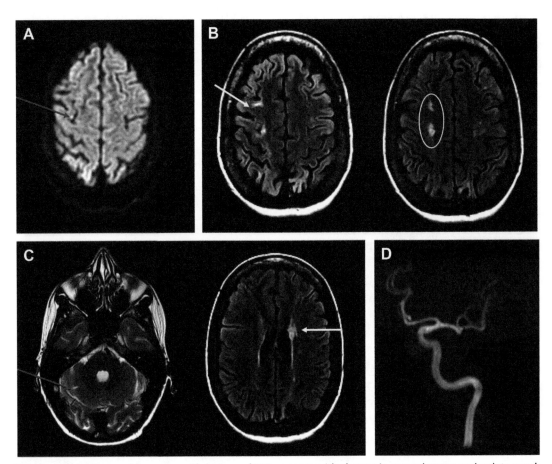

Fig. 14. SLE. A 36-year-old woman with history of SLE presents with change in mental status and palate numbness. (*A*) Axial diffusion-weighted MR image shows punctate acute right frontal cortical infarct (*red arrow*). (*B*) Secondary findings of chronic right frontal subcortical infarct (*yellow arrow*) and white matter lesions paralleling the ventricles (*oval*) on axial T2 FLAIR images are characteristic of lupus. (*C*) Additional chronic infarcts were seen in this young patient, including a chronic right cerebellar infarct on axial T2-weighted MR image (*red arrow*) and left caudate infarct on axial T2 FLAIR-weighted MR image (*yellow arrow*). (*D*) There is a normal appearance of the vessels on 3D MIP image from MRA, which is typical of SLE.

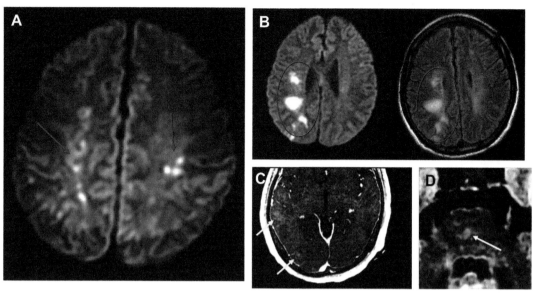

Fig. 15. Intravascular DLBCL. A 54-year-old man presenting with 3 weeks of ascending numbness and malaise, initially treated for Guillain-Barré syndrome. (A) Patient returned for ongoing symptoms, and axial diffusion-weighted MR image revealed multiple bilateral areas of acute infarction in a watershed distribution (red arrows). (B) After 2 months, axial diffusion-weighted and T2 FLAIR images show multiple additional infarcts and infarct-like lesions, with diffusion restriction and corresponding T2 hyperintensity (ovals). (C) Axial T1 postcontrast images revealed leptomeningeal enhancement (yellow arrows). (D) Axial T2 FLAIR shows central pontine T2 hyperintensity (white arrow).

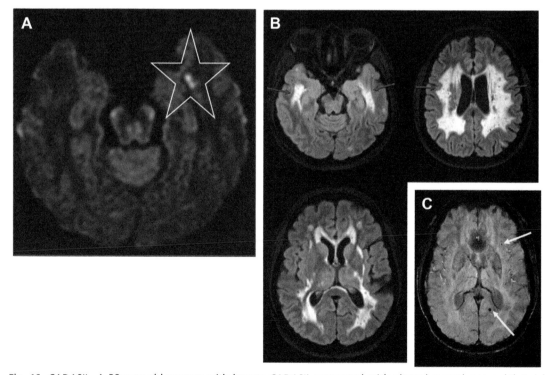

Fig. 16. CADASIL. A 38-year-old woman with known CADASIL presented with altered mental status. (A) Axial diffusion-weighted MR image shows a focus of diffusion restriction in the left temporal subcortical white matter consistent with acute infarct (star). (B) Axial T2 FLAIR images show confluent periventricular white matter hyperintensity involving the anterior temporal and frontal white matter, as well as the external capsule, in a pattern consistent with CADASIL (red arrows). (C) Axial susceptibility-weighted image shows nonspecific microhemorrhages (yellow arrows).

multiple myeloma, T-cell leukemia, and hairy cell leukemia.

There are also hereditary causes of acute infarction. Cerebral autosomal dominant arteriopathy with subcortical infarcts and leukoencephalopathy (CADASIL) causes focal and confluent subcortical white matter infarcts predominantly involving the superior frontal lobes, external capsule, and anterior temporal lobes. Lacunar infarcts and microbleeds may also be seen[35] (**Fig. 16**).

Dissection

Another unusual cause of acute stroke is arterial dissection. This condition often occurs in young patients presenting with focal deficit and headache or neck pain, with a possible inciting event, often trauma. Infarction usually has an embolic cause rather than hypoperfusion.[36,37] Vascular imaging is critical to evaluate for a dissection flap and stenosis or occlusion secondary to dissection. However, in the absence of vascular imaging, a distal cervical ICA dissection may be seen on routine brain MR imaging, so it is important to evaluate the carotid arteries at the skull base for any signs of dissection (**Fig. 17**).

Stroke of Undetermined Cause

This category is invoked when multiple causes or no causes of stroke are identified. Causes that may be missed on conventional cardiac imaging, cardiac work-up, or vascular imaging should be considered as potential causes of cryptogenic stroke. Such entities include patent foramen ovale (**Fig. 18**), aortic arch atherosclerosis, paroxysmal atrial fibrillation,[3] or nonstenosing atherosclerosis of the carotid arteries.[38,39]

HEMORRHAGIC STROKE

Hemorrhagic strokes comprise approximately 5% to 21% of acute strokes.[14] One of the most common causes of hemorrhagic strokes is hypertension.[40] Hypertensive strokes occur in typical locations, including the basal ganglia, thalamus, pons, and cerebellum (**Fig. 19**).

Vascular malformations are another cause of hemorrhagic strokes. Arteriovenous malformations (AVMs) should be considered in younger patients who present with acute hemorrhagic strokes, because hemorrhage is the most common presentation.[41] AVMs are characterized by abnormal arteriovenous connections with a vascular nidus, and absence of an intervening

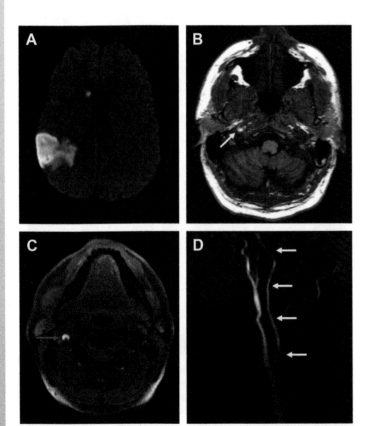

Fig. 17. Cervical carotid dissection. A 40-year-old man with no past medical history presented with acute left facial droop and right jaw pain. (*A*) Axial diffusion-weighted image shows right-sided parietal and caudate head infarcts. (*B*) Axial T1-weighted sequence shows hyperintensity surrounding the right petrous ICA consistent with blood in the dissection flap (*yellow arrow*). (*C*) MRA neck performed for confirmation shows hyperintensity surrounding the proximal cervical ICA on T1 fat-saturated sequence (*red arrow*). (*D*) 3D MRA MIP image shows resultant long segment smooth stenosis extending from just distal to the bifurcation to the petrous ICA (*yellow arrows*).

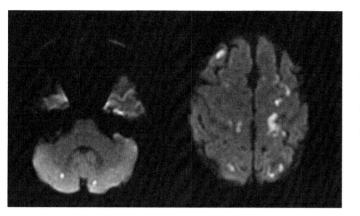

Fig. 18. A 61-year-old-woman with breast cancer and left upper extremity deep venous thrombosis. Axial diffusion-weighted images show multiple bilateral infarctions involving multiple vascular territories. Cause was presumed as secondary to undetected patent foramen ovale, because no large vessel or cardioembolic sources were identified.

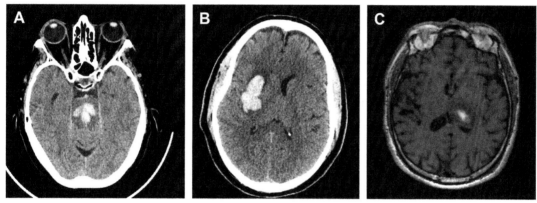

Fig. 19. Three different patients with systemic hypertension, presenting with hemorrhagic infarctions in characteristic locations. In all of these cases, vascular imaging revealed no abnormality. (A) Axial CT with hemorrhagic infarct in the pons. (B) Axial CT with hemorrhagic infarct in the right basal ganglia. (C) Axial T1-weighted MR image with hemorrhagic infarct in the left thalamus.

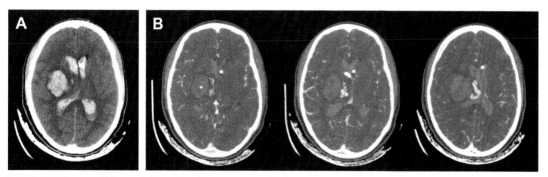

Fig. 20. A 16-year-old boy with no significant past medical history presenting with acute-onset left-sided weakness, headache, and subsequent coma. (A) Axial noncontrast head CT revealed right basal ganglia and intraventricular hemorrhage causing a leftward midline shift. (B) Subsequent CT angiography of the head revealed an arteriovenous malformation with its nidus at the junction between the thalamus and posterior limb of the right internal capsule, supplied by a PCA branch with deep venous drainage.

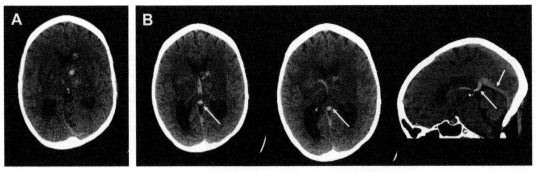

Fig. 21. A 53-year-old woman with history of breast cancer presented after being found down unresponsive. (*A*) Noncontrast head CT at time of presentation shows hemorrhagic infarctions of the bilateral basal ganglia and thalami. (*B*) Tubular hyperdensity is seen in the bilateral internal cerebral veins (*red arrows*), vein of Galen (*yellow arrows*), and straight sinus (*white arrow*), consistent with venous sinus thrombosis and venous infarction.

capillary bed. Vascular imaging with CTA, MRA, or DSA is critical in making the diagnosis (**Fig. 20**).

Venous infarction should be considered when the location of the infarct does not correspond with an arterial vascular distribution, or spans more than 1 arterial distribution (**Fig. 21**). These patients may initially present with vasogenic edema on T2 FLAIR sequences, which, if not addressed, usually progresses to infarction, which

is often hemorrhagic. Secondary findings to search for include presence of a hyperdense venous sinus or cortical vein on noncontrast CT, or absence of flow-related signal void in venous structures on MR imaging. Further evaluation with MR venography or CT venography is often performed for confirmation. Hypercoagulable states are the most important contributing factor in adults.[41,42]

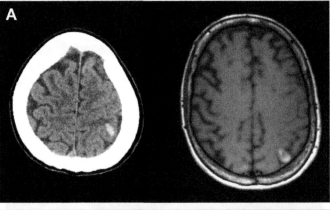

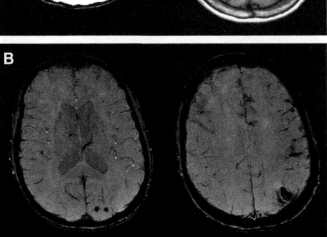

Fig. 22. Cerebral amyloid angiopathy. A 65-year-old woman with recurrent transient neurologic symptoms of unclear cause and migraine with aura, presenting with acute-onset right face and right arm numbness and weakness. (*A*) Axial noncontrast head CT and axial T1-weighted MR image show a left high parietal intraparenchymal hemorrhage. (*B*) Axial susceptibility-weighted images reveal multifocal subarachnoid and subcortical microhemorrhages. Brain biopsy was positive for β-amyloid plaques.

Cerebral amyloid angiopathy is another cause of hemorrhagic infarction to be considered in older patients who present with multiple, recurrent cortical and subcortical hemorrhagic strokes. Susceptibility-weighted imaging is key in making this diagnosis, because multiple foci of parenchymal signal hypointensity are seen in a cortical and subcortical distribution on MR imaging (Fig. 22). Vascular imaging is usually normal.[43]

SUMMARY

Determining the cause of an acute stroke is critical, because this guides patient management. Failure to accurately identify the cause for stroke impairs the clinician's ability to deliver optimal, immediate, acute care and limits the precision with which longer-term therapies can be initiated to prevent stroke recurrence. Patterns on imaging, such as vascular territories affected, vessels involved, and secondary findings, can provide clues to the underlying cause. It is critical to understand these imaging patterns to suggest a cause or recommend further imaging to elucidate the underlying cause. Once large vessel, small vessel, and cardioembolic sources have been excluded, unusual causes should be considered.

ACKNOWLEDGMENTS

Dr. Ajay Gupta's effort is in part supported by NIH grants R01HL14454 and R21HL145427.

REFERENCES

1. Benjamin EJ, Blaha MJ, Chiuve SE, et al. Heart disease and stroke statistics-2017 update: a report from the American Heart Association. Circulation 2017;135(10):e146–603.
2. Yang Q, Tong X, Schieb L, et al. Vital signs: recent trends in stroke death rates - United States, 2000-2015. MMWR Morb Mortal Wkly Rep 2017;66(35): 933–9.
3. Adams HP Jr, Bendixen BH, Kappelle LJ, et al. Classification of subtype of acute ischemic stroke. Definitions for use in a multicenter clinical trial. TOAST. Trial of Org 10172 in acute stroke treatment. Stroke 1993;24(1):35–41.
4. Ay H, Furie KL, Singhal A, et al. An evidence-based causative classification system for acute ischemic stroke. Ann Neurol 2005;58(5):688–97.
5. Chung J-W, Park SH, Kim N, et al. Trial of ORG 10172 in Acute Stroke Treatment (TOAST) classification and vascular territory of ischemic stroke lesions diagnosed by diffusion-weighted imaging. J Am Heart Assoc 2014;3(4):e001119.
6. Derdeyn CP. Mechanisms of ischemic stroke secondary to large artery atherosclerotic disease. Neuroimaging Clin N Am 2007;17(3):303–11, vii–viii.
7. Zimmerman RD. Vascular diseases of the brain. In: Yousem DM, Grossman RI, editors. Neuroradiology: the requisites, vol. 3. Philadelphia: Mosby Elsevier; 2010. p. 104–69.
8. Mattle HP, Arnold M, Lindsberg PJ, et al. Basilar artery occlusion. Lancet Neurol 2011;10(11):1002–14.
9. Kim JS. Pure lateral medullary infarction: clinical–radiological correlation of 130 acute, consecutive patients. Brain 2003;126(8):1864–72.
10. Caplan LR, Hennerici M. Impaired clearance of emboli (washout) is an important link between hypoperfusion, embolism, and ischemic stroke. Arch Neurol 1998;55(11):1475–82.
11. Mangla R, Kolar B, Almast J, et al. Border zone infarcts: pathophysiologic and imaging characteristics. Radiographics 2011;31(5):1201–14.
12. Yong SW, Bang OY, Lee PH, et al. Internal and cortical border-zone infarction: clinical and diffusion-weighted imaging features. Stroke 2006;37(3): 841–6.
13. Belden JR, Caplan LR, Pessin MS, et al. Mechanisms and clinical features of posterior border-zone infarcts. Neurology 1999;53(6):1312–8.
14. Bogousslavsky J, Van Melle G, Regli F. The Lausanne Stroke Registry: analysis of 1,000 consecutive patients with first stroke. Stroke 1988;19(9):1083–92.
15. Depuydt S, Sarov M, Vandendries C, et al. Significance of acute multiple infarcts in multiple cerebral circulations on initial diffusion weighted imaging in stroke patients. J Neurol Sci 2014;337(1–2):151–5.
16. Capmany RP, Ibañez MO, Pesquer XJ. Complex atheromatosis of the aortic arch in cerebral infarction. Curr Cardiol Rev 2010;6(3):184–93.
17. Arboix A, García-Eroles L, Sellarés N, et al. Infarction in the territory of the anterior cerebral artery: clinical study of 51 patients. BMC Neurol 2009;9:30.
18. Bogousslavsky J, Regli F. Anterior cerebral artery territory infarction in the Lausanne Stroke Registry. Clinical and etiologic patterns. Arch Neurol 1990; 47(2):144–50.
19. Kazui S, Sawada T, Naritomi H, et al. Angiographic evaluation of brain infarction limited to the anterior cerebral artery territory. Stroke 1993;24(4):549–53.
20. Kang SY, Kim JS. Anterior cerebral artery infarction: stroke mechanism and clinical-imaging study in 100 patients. Neurology 2008;70(24 Pt 2):2386–93.
21. Arboix A, Arbe G, García-Eroles L, et al. Infarctions in the vascular territory of the posterior cerebral artery: clinical features in 232 patients. BMC Res Notes 2011;4:329.
22. Wardlaw JM, Smith C, Dichgans M. Mechanisms of sporadic cerebral small vessel disease: insights from neuroimaging. Lancet Neurol 2013;12(5): 483–97.

23. Arboix A, Bechich S, Oliveres M, et al. Ischemic stroke of unusual cause: clinical features, etiology and outcome. Eur J Neurol 2001;8(2):133–9.

24. Abdel Razek AA, Alvarez H, Bagg S, et al. Imaging spectrum of CNS vasculitis. Radiographics 2014; 34(4):873–94.

25. Tarasów E, Kułakowska A, Lukasiewicz A, et al. Moyamoya disease: diagnostic imaging. Pol J Radiol 2011;76(1):73–9.

26. Garg A. Vascular brain pathologies. Neuroimaging Clin N Am 2011;21(4):897–926, ix.

27. Tai MS, Viswanathan S, Rahmat K, et al. Cerebral infarction pattern in tuberculous meningitis. Sci Rep 2016;6:38802.

28. Katchanov J, Heuschmann PU, Endres M, et al. Cerebral infarction in bacterial meningitis: predictive factors and outcome. J Neurol 2010;257(5):716–20.

29. Kastenbauer S, Pfister HW. Pneumococcal meningitis in adults: spectrum of complications and prognostic factors in a series of 87 cases. Brain 2003; 126(Pt 5):1015–25.

30. Chiang F, Panyaping T, Tedesqui G, et al. Varicella zoster CNS vascular complications. A report of four cases and literature review. Neuroradiol J 2014;27(3):327–33.

31. Soares BP, Provenzale JM. Imaging of Herpesvirus infections of the CNS. AJR Am J Roentgenol 2016; 206(1):39–48.

32. Lalani TA, Kanne JP, Hatfield GA, et al. Imaging findings in systemic lupus erythematosus. Radiographics 2004;24(4):1069–86.

33. Yamamoto A, Kikuchi Y, Homma K, et al. Characteristics of intravascular large B-cell lymphoma on cerebral MR imaging. AJNR Am J Neuroradiol 2012; 33(2):292–6.

34. Song DK, Boulis NM, McKeever PE, et al. Angiotropic large cell lymphoma with imaging characteristics of CNS vasculitis. AJNR Am J Neuroradiol 2002; 23(2):239–42.

35. Stojanov D, Vojinovic S, Aracki-Trenkic A, et al. Imaging characteristics of cerebral autosomal dominant arteriopathy with subcortical infarcts and leucoencephalopathy (CADASIL). Bosn J Basic Med Sci 2015;15(1):1–8.

36. Benninger DH, Georgiadis D, Kremer C, et al. Mechanism of ischemic infarct in spontaneous carotid dissection. Stroke 2004;35(2):482–5.

37. Lucas C, Moulin T, Deplanque D, et al. Stroke patterns of internal carotid artery dissection in 40 patients. Stroke 1998;29(12):2646–8.

38. Gupta A, Gialdini G, Lerario MP, et al. Magnetic resonance angiography detection of abnormal carotid artery plaque in patients with cryptogenic stroke. J Am Heart Assoc 2015;4(6):e002012.

39. Gupta A, Powers WJ. Nonstenotic carotid plaques: stroke causation or guilt by association? Neurology 2016;87(7):650–1.

40. Hakimi R, Garg A. Imaging of hemorrhagic stroke. Continuum (Minneap Minn) 2016;22(5, Neuroimaging): 1424–50.

41. Heit JJ, Iv M, Wintermark M. Imaging of intracranial hemorrhage. J Stroke 2017;19(1):11–27.

42. Poon CS, Chang J-K, Swarnkar A, et al. Radiologic diagnosis of cerebral venous thrombosis: pictorial review. AJR Am J Roentgenol 2007;189(6_supplement):S64–75.

43. Chao CP, Kotsenas AL, Broderick DF. Cerebral amyloid angiopathy: CT and MR imaging findings. Radiographics 2006;26(5):1517–31.

Perfusion Computed Tomography in Acute Ischemic Stroke

Jeremy J. Heit, MD, PhD[a], Eric S. Sussman, MD[a,b], Max Wintermark, MD[a,*]

KEYWORDS

• Stroke • CT • Perfusion • Core • Penumbra • Infarction • CT angiography

KEY POINTS

- Perfusion CT (PCT) imaging of acute ischemic stroke provides essential information for patient triage to endovascular thrombectomy (EVT).
- PCT delineates the core infarction and ischemic penumbra; patients with a mismatch between these 2 regions are most likely to benefit from EVT.
- PCT may be used to identify and localize large-vessel occlusions.

INTRODUCTION

Acute ischemic stroke (AIS) most commonly results from occlusion of a cerebral or cervical artery, and is the leading cause of disability and fifth leading cause of death in the United States.[1] AIS resulting from arterial occlusions of the internal carotid artery (ICA) and first or second segment of the middle cerebral artery (MCA) are termed large-vessel occlusions (LVOs); these occlusions account for 11% to 29% of AIS cases.[2–4] LVO commonly results in irreversible death of brain tissue, which is termed the core infarction. A variable volume of brain tissue surrounding the core infarction may lack sufficient blood flow to function normally, but often remains viable at the time of presentation. This hypoperfused tissue is termed the penumbra; expeditious restoration of cerebral blood flow may allow for preservation of the penumbra, preventing this tissue from progressing to irreversible infarction. Thus, treatment of the arterial occlusion to restore blood flow to the brain is the primary goal of AIS treatment.

Landmark randomized trials have demonstrated endovascular thrombectomy (EVT) to be an effective treatment of AIS caused by LVO.[5–11] As a result, EVT has become the standard of care in eligible patients.[12] Importantly, diffusion-weighted imaging or perfusion computed tomography (PCT) assessment with clinical mismatch in studies, including the Triage of Wake Up and Late Presenting Strokes Undergoing Neurointervention With Trevo (DAWN)[10] and Endovascular Therapy Following Imaging Evaluation For Ischemic Stroke 3 (DEFUSE 3)[11] trials, demonstrated EVT effectiveness in late time windows (16–24 hours since last seen normal) for patients with favorable neuroimaging profiles. This marked expansion of the AIS treatment window has increased the need for more widespread adoption of advanced neuroimaging to facilitate appropriate triage of AIS patients.

Identification of the core infarction and penumbra in AIS patients using advanced computed tomography (CT) and MR imaging techniques has become an essential component of AIS patient

Disclosures: J.J. Heit: Medtronic, consulting; MicroVention, consulting.
[a] Department of Radiology, Division of Neuroimaging and Neurointervention, Stanford Healthcare, 300 Pasteur Drive, Stanford, CA 94305, USA; [b] Department of Neurosurgery, Stanford Healthcare, 300 Pasteur Drive, Stanford, CA 94305, USA
* Corresponding author. Department of Radiology, Division of Neuroimaging and Neurointervention, Stanford University Hospital, 300 Pasteur Drive, S0047, Stanford, CA 94305.
E-mail address: mwinterm@stanford.edu

Radiol Clin N Am 57 (2019) 1109–1116
https://doi.org/10.1016/j.rcl.2019.06.003
0033-8389/19/© 2019 Elsevier Inc. All rights reserved.

evaluation and EVT triage, particularly in late time windows. Given the widespread availability of CT, PCT is increasingly performed for physiologic evaluation of brain tissue and delineation of core infarction and penumbra.

PCT is performed by injection of an iodinated contrast agent into an antecubital vein, followed by serial imaging of the brain tissue over time. The time-dependent changes in brain density as the iodinated contrast flows through the brain tissue are plotted as a time-density curve, which is used to derive PCT parameter maps.[13] These parameter maps commonly include cerebral blood flow (CBF), cerebral blood volume (CBV), mean transit time (MTT), time to peak (TTP), and the time to maximum (T_{max}) of the residue function. Brain tissue with severely reduced CBV or CBF corresponds to core infarction,[14] and regions of brain with prolongation of the MTT or its derivatives, the TTP or T_{max}, delineate the penumbra (Fig. 1).[14]

This review of PCT for the evaluation of ischemic stroke, with an emphasis on AIS caused by LVO and the use of PCT in EVT triage, begins by briefly reviewing EVT and EVT patient triage using neuroimaging. Readers are referred elsewhere for a discussion of PCT technical details.[13]

ENDOVASCULAR THROMBECTOMY AND IDENTIFICATION OF CANDIDATES FOR ENDOVASCULAR THROMBECTOMY

EVT is an endovascular procedure that mechanically removes arterial thrombus or thromboembolus from a cerebral or cervical artery. Endovascular access is typically obtained via common femoral artery puncture, and endovascular catheters are navigated into the cervical ICA, just proximal to the LVO causing the patient's symptoms. Smaller-diameter catheters are then used to either deploy a stent-retriever device across the occluded vascular segment or apply direct aspiration to the proximal margin of clot, thereby allowing the clot to be mechanically removed from the occluded artery. These newer techniques result in sufficient revascularization of the brain in 59% to 86% of patients and nearly double the likelihood of achieving a good clinical outcome compared with medical therapy alone.[5–11]

Patients who are most likely to benefit from EVT have a specific imaging and clinical profile, which includes (1) an LVO, (2) a relatively small core infarction, and (3) salvageable brain tissue (penumbra) that is greater in size than the core infarction.[15] CT or MR angiography is nearly always performed to identify the presence of an LVO before consideration of EVT.[5–11] However, the manner by which core infarction and penumbra size are determined varies among studies and institutions. The most common ways by which core infarction and penumbra size are assessed are summarized in the following section, with an emphasis on PCT approaches.

CORE INFARCTION DELINEATION AND PERFUSION COMPUTED TOMOGRAPHY FOR CORE INFARCTION VOLUME MEASUREMENT

Diffusion-weighted MR imaging remains the gold standard for the identification of core infarction. However, the more limited availability of MR imaging has led to a reliance on noncontrast CT and PCT-based approaches for core infarction identification and characterization. Noncontrast CT techniques for core infarction delineation include subjective assessment of the extent of brain hypodensity, which is assumed to represent irreversibly infarcted tissue, or the more quantitative 10-point Alberta Stroke Program Early CT Score (ASPECTS).[16] A small core infarction on CT is typically defined as hypodensity that occupies less than one-third of the MCA territory.[5,10,17] By contrast, a small core infarction is typically defined as an ASPECTS of greater than 5[7] or greater than 6.[6,11] ASPECTS is limited by variable inter-rater agreement,[18] but is nonetheless increasingly used to triage AIS patients for EVT treatment, given its relative simplicity and quantitative approach.

Core infarction assessment by PCT may closely approximate the gold standard diffusion-weighted MR imaging,[19–21] although this concept remains controversial.[22–26] Nevertheless, PCT-based approaches to core infarction delineation have been used in several recent randomized EVT trials.[8–11,27] Core infarction on PCT is commonly defined as (1) CBV less than 2.0 to 2.2 mL/100 g, or (2) a relative decrease in CBF by 38% to 70% compared with the contralateral normal hemisphere.[19,21,28–35] Recent positive randomized EVT trials that used PCT-based triage algorithms defined the core infarction as a 70% reduction in CBF relative to the unaffected cerebral hemisphere, and patients with core infarction volumes of less than 20 to 50 mL[8–10] or less than 70 mL[11] were enrolled in these trials. These studies demonstrated a strong treatment benefit of EVT in both early and late time windows. However, the variable core infarction size criteria in these studies have led to further uncertainty as to which patients should be considered for EVT.

Although PCT estimates of core infarction seem to correlate well with diffusion-weighted MR imaging,[32] the accuracy of PCT may be limited in patients presenting within early time windows (ie,

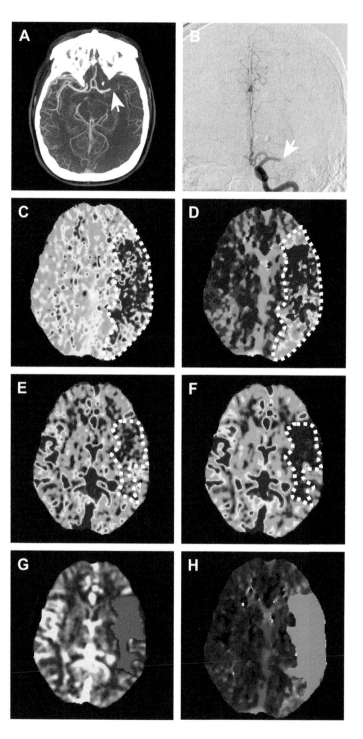

Fig. 1. PCT evaluation of a patient with AIS caused by occlusion of the M1 segment of the left MCA. Occlusion of the left M1 segment is present on axial maximum-intensity projection image CT angiography (*A, arrow*) and digital subtraction angiography (*B, arrow*). PCT (*C–H*) images delineate the penumbra (*C, D, dashed lines*) on MTT (*C*) and T_{max} (*D*) maps. The core infarction (*E, F, dashed lines*) is delineated on CBV (*E*) and CBF (*F*) maps. Quantification of the core infarction (*G, pink*) and penumbra (*H, green*) following automatic processing with RAPID (iSchemaView, Menlo Park, CA).

less than 3 hours since last seen normal). Several studies have found that PCT performed in such cases may overestimate the baseline core infarction in 16% to 38% of patients.[24–26] Overestimation of core infarction by PCT (both CBV and CBF) has been termed the "ghost infarct core"[25,26]; this concept may account for prior studies that found discrepancy between PCT and diffusion-weighted MR imaging measurement of core infarction volumes.[22,36] It is necessary for physicians who treat AIS patients to be cognizant of these potential limitations of using PCT for core infarction delineation.

It is noteworthy that recent randomized EVT trials excluded patients with core infarctions larger than 50 to 70 mL. The strict application of this criterion in clinical practice may exclude a subset of patients who might benefit from EVT treatment. Future randomized trials will determine whether AIS patients with large core infarctions (>50–70 mL) benefit from EVT.[37–39]

PENUMBRA DELINEATION AND PERFUSION COMPUTED TOMOGRAPHY FOR PENUMBRA VOLUME MEASUREMENT

The penumbra is often defined as hypoperfused, but viable brain tissue in patients with AIS caused by LVO,[40] and is assumed to be at risk of irreversible infarction if revascularization of the occluded cerebral artery is not performed.[15] However, this conceptual definition results in some variability in how the volume of penumbra at risk of infarction is measured.

Many neurointerventionalists who treat AIS patients forgo any imaging delineation of the penumbra. These physicians treat patients based on CT, PCT, or MR imaging evidence of a small infarction and a high stroke scale (National Institutes of Health Stroke Scale >6). In these patients, the small size of the core infarction would not entirely explain all of their stroke symptoms, which indicates the presence of a salvageable penumbra. Although this so-called clinical-core mismatch approach for EVT triage has proved to be effective, it is challenging to apply in nonexpert centers.

Many hospitals now routinely perform PCT for the evaluation of AIS patients, as this imaging technique can clearly delineate the penumbra (see **Fig. 1**). The ability to perform PCT at referring primary stroke centers allows for improved detection of patients with AIS caused by LVO who are likely to be EVT candidates.[41,42] Moreover, interhospital relationships and cloud-based image-sharing platforms allow PCT images to be transmitted to neurointerventionalists, neurologists, and radiologists at comprehensive stroke centers, which in turn helps to streamline the interhospital transfer process and facilitate EVT resource mobilization at the accepting facility.

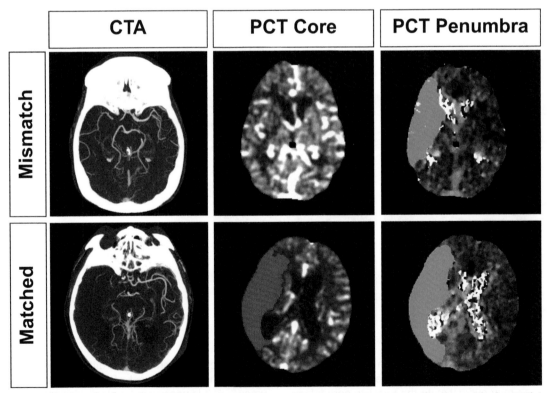

Fig. 2. PCT identification of target mismatch. A patient with a target mismatch profile (favorable for EVT) is shown in the top row. In this patient, CT angiography identifies a right ICA occlusion, and PCT identifies no core infarction and a large penumbra (*green*). A patient with a matched profile (unfavorable for EVT) is shown in the bottom row. In this patient, CT angiography identifies a right ICA occlusion, and PCT identifies a large core infarction (*pink*) and a large penumbra (*green*), which are matched in volume.

On PCT, the penumbra is defined as the difference between the volume of tissue with a specific threshold of hypoperfusion and the core infarction (delineated as described earlier). The penumbra is most commonly defined as MTT prolongation greater than 2.5 to 12 seconds, T_{max} greater than 6 seconds, or decreased CBF.[21,30,33,43,44] These thresholds vary by postprocessing technique, which may introduce significant variability in perfusion maps.[30,44] Therefore, it is essential that each individual center validates their PCT postprocessing software, and maintains consistency in their imaging approach.

PERFUSION COMPUTED TOMOGRAPHY FOR TARGET MISMATCH DELINEATION

Once the core infarction and penumbra are delineated in an AIS patient with an LVO, treating physicians are able to quantitatively and qualitatively compare the relative size of these regions to determine whether a patient is likely to benefit from EVT. Patients who are most likely to benefit from EVT have a mismatch between the core infarction and the penumbra volumes (**Fig. 2**).[8,9,11,15,45] The goal of EVT in these patients is to salvage the penumbra, thereby minimizing the final core infarction volume. Patients with a core infarction volume that

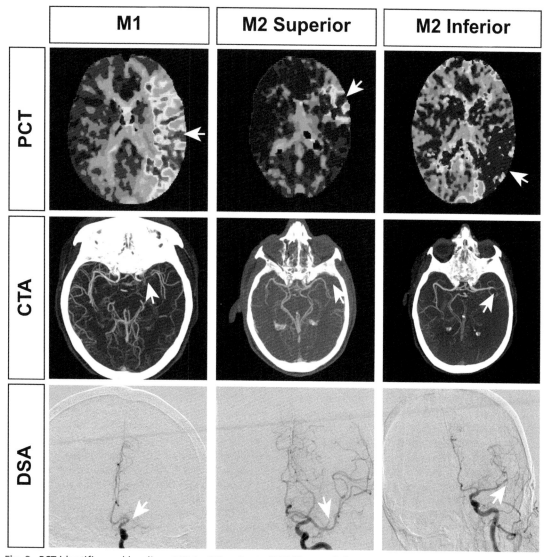

Fig. 3. PCT identifies and localizes LVO in AIS patients. PCT (first row) demonstrates characteristic perfusion deficits (*arrows*) caused by M1 (first column), M2-superior division (second column), and M2-inferior division (third column) occlusions. These LVO locations are confirmed on CT angiography (second row) and digital subtraction angiography (third row).

is matched to the penumbra volume (see **Fig. 2**) are unlikely to benefit from EVT.[15,46] It remains to be determined whether EVT will benefit those patients with large core infarctions (>50–70 mL) with a salvageable penumbra, which is present in up to 17% of patients currently excluded from EVT under current guidelines.[47]

The selective use of EVT for AIS patients with an LVO and mismatch between the volumes of core infarction and penumbra makes intuitive sense, and the application of these criteria to AIS treatment triage should result in superior clinical outcomes after EVT.[15,46] Interestingly, however, a recent meta-analysis found that PCT triage of early-time-window patients did not modify the EVT treatment effect with respect to 90-day clinical outcomes.[48] In this study, small core volume size determined by PCT and patient selection by MR imaging were associated with functional independence at 90 days after treatment. This finding underscores the need for further investigation into how imaging algorithms affect patient outcomes after EVT.[48]

The target mismatch profile on PCT and MR imaging with perfusion MR (PMR) has also been applied to triage AIS patients for intravenous thrombolysis, with promising results.[49–51] It is anticipated that there will be an increase in the use of PCT to select patients for intravenous thrombolysis, particularly in those patients presenting outside of the standard 3- to 4.5-hour window.

PERFUSION COMPUTED TOMOGRAPHY FOR DELINEATION OF LARGE-VESSEL OCCLUSIONS

As detailed earlier, PCT provides important information regarding the volumes of core infarction and penumbra, and the presence of a target mismatch between these volumes. In addition to these essential qualifying characteristics, an AIS patient being considered for EVT must also have an LVO, which is most commonly identified by CT or MR angiography.[5–11] However, LVO presence may also be inferred from PMR or PCT studies (**Fig. 3**).[52,53]

The anatomy of the cerebral arteries and the brain tissue to which they provide blood flow is remarkably consistent in humans. This consistency means that blockage of a specific artery leads to a characteristic perfusion deficit in the brain, which is readily detected by PMR or PCT (see **Fig. 3**). Therefore, the presence of an LVO may be inferred from specific patterns of perfusion deficits on PMR or PCT studies.[52,53] We recently showed that PMR studies viewed in isolation

with MR angiography accurately localize M1-segment MCA occlusions in 96%, and M2-segment MCA occlusions in 90%, of AIS patients.[53] Thus, PCT alone may identify an LVO, while simultaneously providing relevant information regarding core infarction size, penumbra size, and presence of a target mismatch. The identification of all of these imaging characteristics from a single imaging study has the potential to markedly streamline the triage of AIS patients for EVT, particularly if PCT is performed at a referring hospital before transfer to a comprehensive stroke center that offers EVT.

SUMMARY

EVT is a highly effective therapy for AIS caused by LVO. PCT identifies the core infarction volume, penumbra volume, and the presence of a target mismatch between the core and penumbra volumes. In addition, PCT may accurately detect and localize LVOs in AIS patients. Therefore, PCT has become an important tool in the evaluation and triage of AIS patients before EVT. We expect the use of PCT to expand in the near future, as the number of patients who require imaging evaluation to determine EVT candidacy continues to increase.

REFERENCES

1. Mozaffarian D, Benjamin EJ, Go AS, et al. Heart disease and stroke statistics—2015 update: a report from the American Heart Association. Circulation 2015;131(4):e29–322.
2. Rai AT, Seldon AE, Boo S, et al. A population-based incidence of acute large vessel occlusions and thrombectomy eligible patients indicates significant potential for growth of endovascular stroke therapy in the USA. J Neurointerv Surg 2017;9(8):722–6.
3. Go AS, Mozaffarian D, Roger VL, et al. Executive summary: heart disease and stroke statistics—2014 update: a report from the American Heart Association. Circulation 2014;129(3):399–410.
4. Hansen CK, Christensen A, Ovesen C, et al. Stroke severity and incidence of acute large vessel occlusions in patients with hyper-acute cerebral ischemia: results from a prospective cohort study based on CT-angiography (CTA). Int J Stroke 2015;10(3):336–42.
5. Berkhemer OA, Fransen PS, Beumer D, et al. A randomized trial of intraarterial treatment for acute ischemic stroke. N Engl J Med 2015;372(1):11–20.
6. Jovin TG, Chamorro A, Cobo E, et al. Thrombectomy within 8 hours after symptom onset in ischemic stroke. N Engl J Med 2015;372(24):2296–306.

7. Goyal M, Demchuk AM, Menon BK, et al. Randomized assessment of rapid endovascular treatment of ischemic stroke. N Engl J Med 2015;372(11): 1019–30.

8. Saver JL, Goyal M, Bonafe A, et al. Stent-retriever thrombectomy after intravenous t-PA vs. t-PA alone in stroke. N Engl J Med 2015;372(24):2285–95.

9. Campbell BC, Mitchell PJ, Kleinig TJ, et al. Endovascular therapy for ischemic stroke with perfusion-imaging selection. N Engl J Med 2015;372(11): 1009–18.

10. Nogueira RG, Jadhav AP, Haussen DC, et al. Thrombectomy 6 to 24 hours after stroke with a mismatch between deficit and infarct. N Engl J Med 2018; 378(1):11–21.

11. Albers GW, Marks MP, Kemp S, et al. Thrombectomy for stroke at 6 to 16 hours with selection by perfusion imaging. N Engl J Med 2018;378(8): 708–18.

12. Powers WJ, Rabinstein AA, Ackerson T, et al. 2018 guidelines for the early management of patients with acute ischemic stroke: a guideline for healthcare professionals from the American Heart Association/American Stroke Association. Stroke 2018; 49(3):e46–110.

13. Heit JJ, Wintermark M. Perfusion computed tomography for the evaluation of acute ischemic stroke: strengths and pitfalls. Stroke 2016;47(4): 1153–8.

14. Wintermark M, Albers GW, Alexandrov AV, et al. Acute stroke imaging research roadmap. Stroke 2008;39(5):1621–8.

15. Heit JJ, Wintermark M. Imaging selection for reperfusion therapy in acute ischemic stroke. Curr Treat Options Neurol 2015;17(2):332.

16. Barber PA, Demchuk AM, Zhang J, et al. Validity and reliability of a quantitative computed tomography score in predicting outcome of hyperacute stroke before thrombolytic therapy. ASPECTS Study Group. Alberta Stroke Programme Early CT Score. Lancet 2000;355(9216):1670–4.

17. The National Institute of Neurological Disorders and Stroke rt-PA Stroke Study Group. Tissue plasminogen activator for acute ischemic stroke. N Engl J Med 1995;333(24):1581–7.

18. Gupta AC, Schaefer PW, Chaudhry ZA, et al. Interobserver reliability of baseline noncontrast CT Alberta Stroke Program Early CT Score for intraarterial stroke treatment selection. AJNR Am J Neuroradiol 2012;33(6):1046–9.

19. Campbell BC, Christensen S, Levi CR, et al. Cerebral blood flow is the optimal CT perfusion parameter for assessing infarct core. Stroke 2011;42(12): 3435–40.

20. Donahue J, Wintermark M. Perfusion CT and acute stroke imaging: foundations, applications, and literature review. J Neuroradiol 2015;42(1):21–9.

21. Wintermark M, Flanders AE, Velthuis B, et al. Perfusion-CT assessment of infarct core and penumbra: receiver operating characteristic curve analysis in 130 patients suspected of acute hemispheric stroke. Stroke 2006;37(4):979–85.

22. Copen WA, Morais LT, Wu O, et al. In acute stroke, can CT perfusion-derived cerebral blood volume maps substitute for diffusion-weighted imaging in identifying the ischemic core? PLoS One 2015; 10(7):e0133566.

23. Copen WA, Yoo AJ, Rost NS, et al. In patients with suspected acute stroke, CT perfusion-based cerebral blood flow maps cannot substitute for DWI in measuring the ischemic core. PLoS One 2017; 12(11):e0188891.

24. Silvennoinen HM, Hamberg LM, Lindsberg PJ, et al. CT perfusion identifies increased salvage of tissue in patients receiving intravenous recombinant tissue plasminogen activator within 3 hours of stroke onset. AJNR Am J Neuroradiol 2008;29(6):1118–23.

25. Boned S, Padroni M, Rubiera M, et al. Admission CT perfusion may overestimate initial infarct core: the ghost infarct core concept. J Neurointerv Surg 2017;9(1):66–9.

26. Martins N, Aires A, Mendez B, et al. Ghost infarct core and admission computed tomography perfusion: redefining the role of neuroimaging in acute ischemic stroke. Interv Neurol 2018;7(6):513–21.

27. Kidwell CS, Jahan R, Gornbein J, et al. A trial of imaging selection and endovascular treatment for ischemic stroke. N Engl J Med 2013;368(10): 914–23.

28. Bivard A, Levi C, Spratt N, et al. Perfusion CT in acute stroke: a comprehensive analysis of infarct and penumbra. Radiology 2013;267(2):543–50.

29. McVerry F, Dani KA, MacDougall NJ, et al. Derivation and evaluation of thresholds for core and tissue at risk of infarction using CT perfusion. J Neuroimaging 2014;24(6):562–8.

30. Kamalian S, Kamalian S, Konstas AA, et al. CT perfusion mean transit time maps optimally distinguish benign oligemia from true "at-risk" ischemic penumbra, but thresholds vary by postprocessing technique. AJNR Am J Neuroradiol 2012;33(3): 545–9.

31. Wintermark M, Reichhart M, Thiran JP, et al. Prognostic accuracy of cerebral blood flow measurement by perfusion computed tomography, at the time of emergency room admission, in acute stroke patients. Ann Neurol 2002;51(4):417–32.

32. Cereda CW, Christensen S, Campbell BC, et al. A benchmarking tool to evaluate computer tomography perfusion infarct core predictions against a DWI standard. J Cereb Blood Flow Metab 2016;36(10): 1780–9.

33. Qiao Y, Zhu G, Patrie J, et al. Optimal perfusion computed tomographic thresholds for ischemic

core and penumbra are not time dependent in the clinically relevant time window. Stroke 2014;45(5): 1355–62.

34. Angermaier A, Khaw AV, Kirsch M, et al. Influence of recanalization and time of cerebral ischemia on tissue outcome after endovascular stroke treatment on computed tomography perfusion. J Stroke Cerebrovasc Dis 2015;24(10):2306–12.

35. Bivard A, Levi C, Krishnamurthy V, et al. Defining acute ischemic stroke tissue pathophysiology with whole brain CT perfusion. J Neuroradiol 2014; 41(5):307–15.

36. Schaefer PW, Souza L, Kamalian S, et al. Limited reliability of computed tomographic perfusion acute infarct volume measurements compared with diffusion-weighted imaging in anterior circulation stroke. Stroke 2015;46(2):419–24.

37. Rebello LC, Bouslama M, Haussen DC, et al. Endovascular treatment for patients with acute stroke who have a large ischemic core and large mismatch imaging profile. JAMA Neurol 2017;74(1):34–40.

38. Yoo AJ, Berkhemer OA, Fransen PSS, et al. Effect of baseline Alberta Stroke Program Early CT Score on safety and efficacy of intra-arterial treatment: a subgroup analysis of a randomised phase 3 trial (MR CLEAN). Lancet Neurol 2016;15(7):685–94.

39. Goyal M, Almekhlafi MA, Cognard C, et al. Which patients with acute stroke due to proximal occlusion should not be treated with endovascular thrombectomy? Neuroradiology 2018;61(1):3–8.

40. Astrup J, Siesjo BK, Symon L. Thresholds in cerebral ischemia—the ischemic penumbra. Stroke 1981; 12(6):723–5.

41. Aghaebrahim A, Sauvageau E, Aguilar-Salinas P, et al. Referral facility CT perfusion prior to inter-facility transfer in patients undergoing mechanical thrombectomy. J Neurointerv Surg 2018;10(9):818–22.

42. Guenego A, Mlynash M, Christensen S, et al. Hypoperfusion ratio predicts infarct growth during transfer for thrombectomy. Ann Neurol 2018;84(4): 616–20.

43. Carrera E, Jones PS, Iglesias S, et al. The vascular mean transit time: a surrogate for the penumbra flow threshold? J Cereb Blood Flow Metab 2011; 31(4):1027–35.

44. Maija R, Gaida K, Karlis K, et al. Perfusion computed tomography relative threshold values in definition of acute stroke lesions. Acta Radiol Short Rep 2013; 2(3). 2047981613486099.

45. Baron JC, von Kummer R, del Zoppo GJ. Treatment of acute ischemic stroke. Challenging the concept of a rigid and universal time window. Stroke 1995; 26(12):2219–21.

46. Albers GW. Late window paradox. Stroke 2018; 49(3):768–71.

47. Bahr Hosseini M, Woolf G, Sharma LK, et al. The frequency of substantial salvageable penumbra in thrombectomy-ineligible patients with acute stroke. J Neuroimaging 2018;28(6):676–82.

48. Campbell BCV, Majoie C, Albers GW, et al. Penumbral imaging and functional outcome in patients with anterior circulation ischaemic stroke treated with endovascular thrombectomy versus medical therapy: a meta-analysis of individual patient-level data. Lancet Neurol 2019;18(1):46–55.

49. Hacke W, Furlan AJ, Al-Rawi Y, et al. Intravenous desmoteplase in patients with acute ischaemic stroke selected by MRI perfusion-diffusion weighted imaging or perfusion CT (DIAS-2): a prospective, randomised, double-blind, placebo-controlled study. Lancet Neurol 2009;8(2):141–50.

50. Kate M, Wannamaker R, Kamble H, et al. Penumbral imaging-based thrombolysis with tenecteplase is feasible up to 24 hours after symptom onset. J Stroke 2018;20(1):122–30.

51. Campbell BCV, Mitchell PJ, Churilov L, et al. Tenecteplase versus alteplase before thrombectomy for ischemic stroke. N Engl J Med 2018;378(17): 1573–82.

52. Staroselskaya IA, Chaves C, Silver B, et al. Relationship between magnetic resonance arterial patency and perfusion-diffusion mismatch in acute ischemic stroke and its potential clinical use. Arch Neurol 2001;58(7):1069–74.

53. Wolman DN, Iv M, Wintermark M, et al. Can diffusion- and perfusion-weighted imaging alone accurately triage anterior circulation acute ischemic stroke patients to endovascular therapy? J Neurointerv Surg 2018;10(12):1132–6.

Central Nervous System Vasculopathies

Jennifer E. Soun, MD[a],*, Jae W. Song, MD, MS[b], Javier M. Romero, MD[c],
Pamela W. Schaefer, MD[c]

KEYWORDS

- Central nervous system • Vasculopathy • Vasculitis • Brain imaging

KEY POINTS

- CNS vasculopathies comprise a heterogeneous group of disorders with multiple different causes, including noninflammatory and inflammatory etiologies.
- Distinguishing salient clinical and imaging features helps with diagnosis and initiation of appropriate treatment.
- Imaging techniques, including advanced MR sequences, in conjunction with the clinical presentation and laboratory markers, play an important role in diagnosis and management of these disorders.

INTRODUCTION

Central nervous system (CNS) vasculopathies are challenging to diagnose because of the wide spectrum of disorders. Various causes have been described, including idiopathic, inflammatory, infectious, drug-induced, iatrogenic, connective tissue disorders, and gene mutations.[1,2] For the vasculopathies attributable to vasculitis, or inflammation of the vessel wall, the 2012 Revised International Chapel Hill Consensus Conference Nomenclature of Vasculitides provides a framework for organization based on the size of the involved vessel or on single-organ involvement, systemic involvement, or probable cause.[3] Patient demographics, clinical presentation, other organ involvement, serum and cerebrospinal fluid markers, and neuroimaging play an important role in diagnosis and management. This article provides an overview of the salient clinical and imaging features of noninflammatory and inflammatory CNS vasculopathies.

IMAGING TECHNIQUES

Various imaging techniques are used to diagnose CNS vasculopathies. A noncontrast head computed tomography (CT) scan can detect macrohemorrhage or infarction. MR diffusion-weighted imaging (DWI) and susceptibility-weighted imaging (SWI) show acute infarctions and microhemorrhages, respectively. T2-weighted and fluid-attenuation inversion recovery (FLAIR) sequences demonstrate changes in white matter, and postcontrast images detect blood-brain barrier breakdown, which can manifest as abnormal leptomeningeal, dural, or parenchymal enhancement. CT angiography (CTA) and MR angiography (MRA) are used to evaluate luminal irregularity, narrowing, occlusion, or aneurysm. However, MRA may overestimate the degree of narrowing and is less sensitive in distal vessels.[4] Color Doppler ultrasonography can evaluate extracranial vessel wall thickening and degree of stenoses.[5] 18F-labeled fluorodeoxyglucose (FDG) PET/CT has a role in diagnosing extracranial and

Disclosure Statement: The authors have nothing to disclose.
[a] Department of Radiological Sciences, University of California, Irvine, 101 The City Drive South, Orange, CA 92868, USA; [b] Department of Radiology, Division of Neuroradiology, University of Pennsylvania, 3400 Spruce Street, Philadelphia, PA 19104, USA; [c] Department of Neuroradiology, Massachusetts General Hospital, Harvard Medical School, 55 Fruit Street, Boston, MA 02114, USA
* Corresponding author.
E-mail address: jesoun@uci.edu
; @jsongmd (J.W.S.)

radiologic.theclinics.com

systemic vasculopathy findings. Digital subtraction angiography (DSA) is considered the imaging gold standard for diagnosing most vasculopathies because it has the highest spatial resolution and can identify culprit vascular lesions when noninvasive imaging is negative.[6,7]

Newer advanced imaging techniques are also being used to evaluate vasculopathies. Vessel wall imaging (VWI) is a black-blood MR imaging technique with blood and CSF suppression allowing visualization of vessel wall pathology to help distinguish among different intracranial vasculopathies.[8] Recent studies have also shown that VWI can identify vessels with abnormal wall enhancement for targeted biopsy.[9] When imaging methods are nonspecific, biopsy is sometimes required.

IMAGING FEATURES OF CENTRAL NERVOUS SYSTEM VASCULOPATHIES
Noninflammatory Vasculopathies

Atheromatous disease
Atherosclerotic disease comprises the vast majority of noninflammatory vasculopathies and affects both intracranial and extracranial vessels. Although this entity is not discussed in detail here, it is important to remember that atherosclerosis can occur in conjunction with or mimic other CNS vasculopathies. Vessel involvement favors proximal intracranial and cervical arteries. Although there can be an overlap, vessel wall involvement tends to be eccentric and focal rather than concentric and segmental as seen in vasculitis (**Fig. 1**).[10]

Cerebral autosomal dominant arteriopathy with subcortical infarcts and leukoencephalopathy
Cerebral autosomal dominant arteriopathy with subcortical infarcts and leukoencephalopathy (CADASIL) is a nonatherosclerotic, nonamyloid genetic vasculopathy affecting small cerebral vessels caused by a notch3 mutation.[11] Patients often present in adulthood (mean age of onset 41–49 years old) with recurrent subcortical strokes, dementia, migraines with aura, pseudobulbar palsy, and psychiatric disturbances.[11] Distinguishing imaging features include periventricular and subcortical white matter involvement, notably in the anterior temporal lobes and external capsules (**Fig. 2**).[11] Microbleeds are commonly present in symptomatic patients, with predilection for the thalami, brainstem, white matter, and cortical-subcortical regions, but they can have a widespread distribution.[12,13]

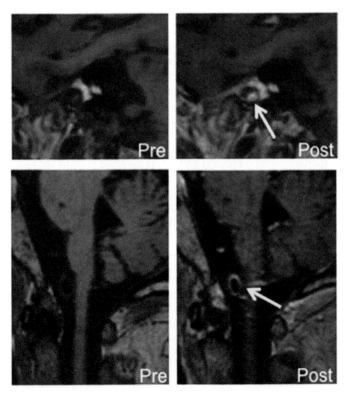

Fig. 1. Vessel wall imaging for atherosclerosis (*top*) and vasculitis (*bottom*). Top: eccentric wall thickening and heterogeneous enhancement (*arrow*) is present in the intracranial internal carotid artery, characteristic for atherosclerosis. Bottom: circumferential wall thickening and enhancement (*arrow*) is more characteristic of an inflammatory vasculitis, as seen in the basilar artery of this patient with primary angiitis of the CNS.

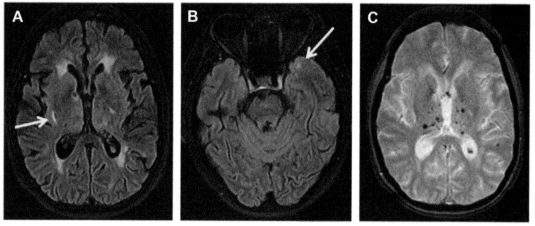

Fig. 2. A patient with CADASIL with characteristic hyperintense white matter lesions in the external capsule (*A, arrow*) and anterior temporal lobe (*B, arrow*) on FLAIR images. Gradient echo (GRE) images (*C*) show microhemorrhages, predominantly in the thalami.

Susac syndrome

Susac syndrome is a microangiopathy of unknown pathogenesis that affects the brain, retina, and cochlea.[14] Patients are typically women in their twenties to forties. The classic clinical triad includes encephalopathy, visual deficit from branch retinal artery occlusions, and sensorineural hearing loss.[14] Imaging features include white matter lesions with variable enhancement and callosal lesions involving the central fibers with a T2/FLAIR-hyperintense and T1-hypointense "snowball" appearance (**Fig. 3**).[14,15] Distinguishing MR features of Susac syndrome and multiple sclerosis are listed in **Table 1**.[15]

Moyamoya

Moyamoya is a progressive steno-occlusive vasculopathy that can be idiopathic (moyamoya disease [MMD]) or related to conditions (moyamoya syndrome) such as atherosclerosis, Down syndrome, sickle cell anemia, neurofibromatosis type 1, radiation, connective tissue disorders, or infection. Children often present with ischemic infarction in borderzone or subcortical areas, whereas adults often present with hemorrhagic infarctions.[16]

Typical vessel involvement includes narrowing of the terminal internal carotid and proximal anterior and middle cerebral arteries, with rare involvement of the posterior circulation (**Fig. 4**).[16,17] Patients develop fragile collaterals, which cause the "puff-of-smoke" appearance on vessel imaging. On FLAIR, leptomeningeal hyperintense signal, termed the "ivy sign," reflects slow flow via leptomeningeal anastomoses.[18] Postcontrast MR images demonstrate corresponding leptomeningeal enhancement. DSA allows preoperative assessment of anastomoses

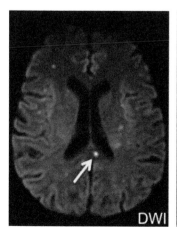
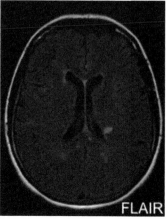

Fig. 3. A 59-year-old woman with Susac syndrome with headache, branch retinal artery occlusion, and hearing loss. MR imaging shows scattered punctate FLAIR-hyperintense white matter lesions, some of which have restricted diffusion. A callosal lesion (*arrow*) has the typical "snowball" appearance.

Table 1
Comparison of MR imaging findings for Susac syndrome and multiple sclerosis

Susac Syndrome	Multiple Sclerosis
Punctate white matter lesions	Ovoid white matter lesions
Central callosal lesions	Peripheral callosal or callososeptal lesions
Leptomeningeal enhancement	No leptomeningeal enhancement
No spinal cord lesions	Spinal cord lesions

and evaluation of post-revascularization collaterals.[16] Perfusion imaging helps monitor blood flow changes after revascularization.[19] Microbleeds occur in up to 30% of Asian patients and are associated with an increased risk of hemorrhagic stroke.[20] Incidental aneurysms occur in 3.6% of adults with nonhemorrhagic MMD.[16,21] Treatment involves bypassing the occluded segments with direct, indirect, or combined revascularization techniques.

Fibromuscular dysplasia

Fibromuscular dysplasia (FMD) is a medium-vessel vasculopathy most commonly affecting middle-aged Caucasian women. Typical clinical presentations include headache, dizziness, and pulsatile tinnitus.[22,23] The most common vessel involved is the renal artery (79.7%), followed closely by the extracranial internal carotid artery (74.3%) and the vertebral artery (36.6%).[24] The 2014 American Heart Association (AHA) recommendations classify the disease into multifocal (most commonly medial fibroplasia) and focal (most commonly intimal fibroplasia) subtypes.[22,23] Complications include dissection, stenosis, occlusion, or aneurysm rupture.

Because of the higher prevalence of intracranial aneurysms in FMD patients compared with the general population, the AHA recommends one-time screening.[22,23] Treatment typically includes antiplatelet therapy and treatment of complications.[23]

The classic vessel imaging appearance on DSA and CTA is a "string of beads" with alternating stenosis and dilatation (**Fig. 5**). Ultrasonography can evaluate the cervical vessels for abnormal flow-related disturbances but is limited in evaluating vessels at the skull base or intracranially.[22,23] Other vessel imaging findings include tortuosity, dissection, stenosis/occlusions, or aneurysms.

Carotid web

Carotid webs are likely secondary to focal FMD, affecting the vessel wall intima rather than media, and are associated with cryptogenic stroke in young patients.[25,26] CTA is the best noninvasive imaging technique for detecting a carotid web, which appears as a shelf-like intraluminal defect along the posterior wall of the carotid bulb (**Fig. 6**).[26] No standard treatment guidelines exist, but recent studies suggest that surgical revascularization of the carotid artery is better than medical management for preventing recurrent strokes.[25]

Vasculopathy associated with connective tissue disorders

Connective tissue disorders, including Marfan syndrome, Ehlers-Danlos syndrome type IV, and Loeys-Dietz syndrome (LDS), are caused by genetic defects that impair connective tissue, resulting in weakened vessel walls.[27] These disorders are autosomal dominant, but sporadic mutations can occur.[27] Marfan syndrome is caused by a defect in the fibrillin-1 gene, which results in aortic root dilatation or dissection, ectopia lentis, musculoskeletal involvement, and dural ectasia.[1,28]

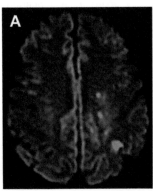
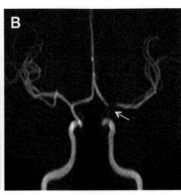

Fig. 4. A patient with moyamoya syndrome with left-sided borderzone infarctions on DWI (*A*) and severe narrowing of the left intracranial internal carotid artery terminus and origins of the left anterior and middle cerebral arteries (*B, arrow*).

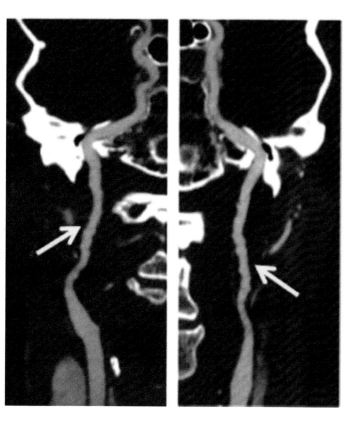

Fig. 5. A 60-year-old woman with fibromuscular dysplasia shows marked beading (*arrows*) of both distal cervical internal carotid arteries.

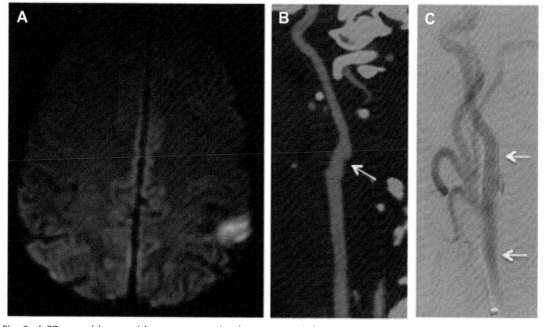

Fig. 6. A 37-year-old man with recurrent strokes has an acute left postcentral gyrus infarction on DWI (*A*) and a carotid web on CTA (*B, arrow*). Subsequently, a stent was placed in the internal carotid artery (*C, arrows*).

Ehlers-Danlos type IV is caused by a defect in the COL3A1 gene that encodes for type III collagen, with manifestations of skin translucency, arterial or visceral rupture, extensive bruising, characteristic facial appearance, and cavernous-carotid fistulas.[27,29] LDS is caused by mutations in the transforming growth factor β signaling pathway, with a clinical triad of hypertelorism, a bifid uvula or cleft palate, and arterial tortuosity with aneurysms and dissections.[30] Aortic root aneurysms and intracranial aneurysms are commonly seen in these entities.[27,31]

Surveillance with vessel imaging is important, as arterial dissections and aneurysm ruptures significantly contribute to morbidity and mortality.[1,31] Tortuosity (**Fig. 7**) and friability of vessels make endovascular treatments challenging and are only reserved for symptomatic patients.

Reversible cerebral vasoconstrictive syndrome

Reversible cerebral vasoconstrictive syndrome (RCVS) is associated with exposure to various vasoactive triggers and is characterized by thunderclap headaches and reversibility of angiographic findings.[32–36] RCVS is considered self-limiting with a favorable outcome, but causes significant morbidity in less than 5% of patients.[35]

CT or MR imaging findings of RCVS include convexity subarachnoid hemorrhage, vasogenic edema (posterior reversible encephalopathy syndrome [PRES]), infarctions, or parenchymal hemorrhage.[32,34,36,37] PRES is detected as confluent subcortical T2/FLAIR-hyperintense white matter changes and is seen in 8% to 38% of patients.[34,35] Vessel imaging shows reversible segmental arterial narrowing appearing as a "string of beads" or "sausage on a string" (**Fig. 8**).[32,33,35,36] Transcranial Doppler ultrasonography can monitor vasoconstriction by measuring blood flow velocities.[37] Studies suggest VWI may help distinguish RCVS from inflammatory CNS vasculitides because RCVS demonstrates more diffuse uniform wall thickening and less wall enhancement.[8,37] In studies comparing RCVS and primary angiitis of the CNS (PACNS), the features of either (1) recurrent thunderclap headaches or (2) single thunderclap headache in combination with normal imaging, borderzone infarctions, or PRES had a 100% positive predictive value for diagnosing RCVS.[32,36] Unlike PACNS, RCVS sometimes presents with normal MR imaging despite vasoconstriction.[32,36] **Table 2** compares RCVS with PACNS.

Inflammatory Vasculopathies

Large-vessel vasculitis

Takayasu arteritis Takayasu arteritis (TAK) is a chronic large-vessel inflammatory vasculitis involving the aorta and its main branches and pulmonary arteries (**Fig. 9**).[1] TAK typically affects women in the second or third decade.[3,16,38] Vessel wall inflammation and later intimal proliferation and fibrosis cause narrowing, occlusion, dilatation, and aneurysm formation.[2]

There are two phases of TAK. In the early phase, patients present with constitutional systems and vascular pain.[16,38] In the late phase, ischemic symptoms develop, including

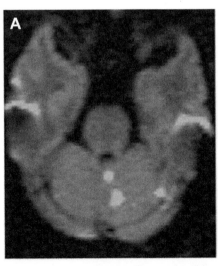
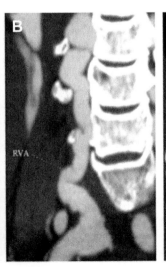
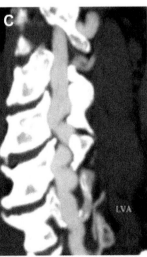

Fig. 7. A 50-year-old man with vascular Ehlers-Danlos type IV with dizziness. Imaging shows acute infarctions in the cerebellum (*A*) and tortuosity with multifocal dilatation of the vertebral arteries (*B, C*).

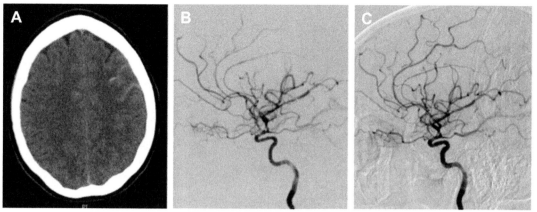

Fig. 8. A 39-year-old woman with reversible cerebral vasoconstrictive syndrome with thunderclap headache in the setting of selective serotonin reuptake inhibitor and marijuana use. CT shows left frontal convexity subarachnoid hemorrhage (*A*). DSA shows diffuse multifocal narrowing of the anterior and middle cerebral arteries (*B*), which improves after administration of intra-arterial verapamil (*C*).

claudication, syncope, hypertension, bruits, diminished pulses, and blood pressure discrepancy.[38,39] CTA and MRA have high sensitivity and specificity (>90%) for diagnosing TAK, whereas Doppler ultrasonography has high specificity but lower sensitivity (81% in a meta-analysis).[40,41] Multiple imaging modalities have shown mixed results in monitoring disease

Table 2
Comparison of reversible cerebral vasoconstrictive syndrome and primary angiitis of the central nervous system

	RCVS	PACNS
Clinical presentation	Thunderclap headache in young women	Insidious headache, cognitive impairment in middle-aged men
Triggers	Vasoconstrictive medications (sympathomimetics, serotonergic antidepressants), illicit drugs (cocaine, amphetamines, marijuana), pregnancy/postpartum state, and physiologic triggers (sexual activity, Valsalva)	None
CSF findings	Normal	Lymphocytic pleocytosis, elevated total protein
Histologic findings	Normal	Granulomatous, lymphocytic, or necrotizing vasculitis
Imaging findings	• Reversible after 3 months • Segmental arterial narrowing • Borderzone infarctions • Convexity subarachnoid hemorrhage • PRES	• Variable duration, depends on severity • Variable focal or multifocal segmental arterial narrowing • Variable location of infarctions, including deep gray and white matter • Parenchymal hemorrhage
Treatment	Remove offending agent, calcium-channel blockers	Steroids, cytotoxic therapy

Abbreviations: CSF, cerebrospinal fluid; PACNS, primary angiitis of the central nervous system; PRES, posterior reversible encephalopathy syndrome; RCVS, reversible cerebral vasoconstrictive syndrome.

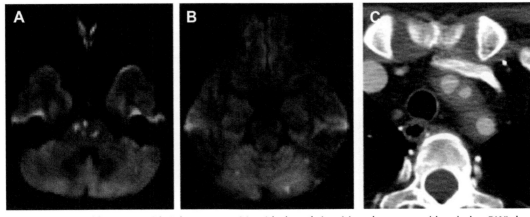

Fig. 9. A 36-year-old woman with Takayasu arteritis with dysarthria, vision changes, and headache. DWI shows acute pontine and cerebellar infarctions (*A, B*). CTA shows circumferential soft-tissue thickening of the aortic arch and origins of the great vessels (*C*).

activity and response to therapy.[10,16,40,41] DSA is helpful in showing stenoses, occlusions, collaterals, subclavian steal phenomenon, and for endovascular intervention.[39,40] Vessel wall thickening and enhancement on MR imaging in the early phase correlates with elevated inflammatory markers.[42] Vessel wall edema on T2-weighted MR sequences and increased carotid artery intima-to-media thickness on ultrasonography may also be markers of active inflammation.[2,41]

Giant cell arteritis Giant cell arteritis (GCA) is a chronic, immune-mediated inflammatory vasculitis of large and medium-sized vessels, most commonly involving external carotid artery branches and the thoracic aorta and its branches in women older than 50 years.[1,3] Histologically, GCA is indistinguishable from TAK, and some consider both entities as part of the same disease spectrum.[3] Patients often present with temporal arteritis and a coexisting polymyalgia rheumatica.[16,43] Symptoms include jaw claudication, temporal headaches, vision loss, scalp tenderness, and elevated inflammatory markers.[1,16]

CTA and MRA show vessel wall thickening, stenoses, and occlusions, most commonly of the superficial temporal artery. Ultrasonography shows a hypoechoic, thickened superficial temporal artery wall, the "halo sign," which aids diagnosis and disease activity surveillance during therapy.[44] In challenging cases, biopsy is required.[2,5,16,44] FDG PET has a role in diagnosing inflammation of extracranial vessels, but its efficacy during treatment is less clear.[43] VWI can be accurate in the initial diagnosis of superficial temporal artery involvement in GCA.[45] As in TAK, monitoring disease activity and treatment effect with imaging has produced varying results and remains under investigation.[40,43]

Medium-vessel vasculitis
Polyarteritis nodosa Polyarteritis nodosa is an antineutrophil cytoplasmic antibodies (ANCA)-negative necrotizing vasculitis of medium and small vessels that typically affects renal arteries in older males.[3] Rare CNS vessel involvement includes aneurysms, stenosis, or occlusions.[2] Because medium and small vessels are most commonly affected, infarctions are typically cortical or subcortical.[46]

Kawasaki disease Kawasaki disease, or mucocutaneous lymph node syndrome, is a vasculitis of medium and small vessels affecting infants and young children.[3,47] The clinical findings include fever for at least 5 days, extremity erythema or edema, polymorphous exanthema, painless bulbar conjunctival injection, oral cavity erythema, strawberry tongue, cervical lymphadenopathy, and coronary artery aneurysms.[47] Rare CNS imaging findings include transient subcortical FLAIR-hyperintense lesions, subdural effusions, infarctions, reversible splenial lesions, and parenchymal atrophy.[2,48]

Small-vessel vasculitis
Small-vessel vasculitides are categorized by vessel wall immunoglobulin deposition: ANCA-associated (none or few deposits) and immune complex (many deposits).[3] CNS involvement is -uncommon and includes vessel irregularities, pachymeningitis, infarctions, hemorrhage, T2-hyperintense lesions, PRES, hypophyseal involvement, and transverse myelitis.[2,49–52] Granulomas in granulomatosis with polyangiitis can be isolated or secondary to direct extension from the orbits or sinonasal cavities.[2] Peripheral neuropathy and

cranial nerve involvement can be seen in any of these entities.[2,49,50]

Variable-vessel vasculitis

Behçet disease Behçet disease is a relapsing multisystem disease of unknown cause, typically presenting with oral and genital ulcers and uveitis.[53,54] There are two main subtypes of neuro-Behçet, parenchymal and nonparenchymal. The parenchymal subtype is more common and considered an inflammatory meningoencephalitis, whereas the nonparenchymal subtype results from vascular involvement.[54]

Parenchymal neuro-Behçet manifests as enhancing T2-hyperintense lesions in the brainstem and to a lesser extent involving the basal ganglia, thalami, cerebral hemispheres, spinal cord, and cranial nerves (**Fig. 10**).[53,54] Classic brainstem lesions involve the pons and cerebral peduncles.[53] Lesions can show restricted diffusion in the acute phase and atrophy in the chronic phase.[54] Nonparenchymal neuro-Behçet imaging findings include aseptic meningitis, venous sinus thrombosis, dissection, occlusion,

infarction, or aneurysm.[2,53,54] Occasionally the lesions are mass-like, mimicking tumors or abscesses.[53,55]

Single-organ vasculitis

Primary angiitis of the central nervous system PACNS is a vasculitis affecting medium- and small-sized vessels without systemic involvement. PACNS most commonly affects 40- to 60-year-old men and presents with nonspecific symptoms such as insidious headache or cognitive impairment.[56,57] Three vasculitic patterns include granulomatous, necrotizing, and lymphocytic types.[58] Treatment is with steroids and cytotoxic agents.[56]

PACNS has imaging features that overlap with many noninflammatory and inflammatory vasculopathies, thromboembolic diseases, demyelinating disease, infection, and neoplasms.[32,56,57] Vessel imaging typically shows variable focal or multifocal segmental narrowing. However, the absence of pathology on vessel imaging does not exclude the diagnosis. MR imaging often shows multifocal infarctions and predominantly subcortical white matter lesions, although deep

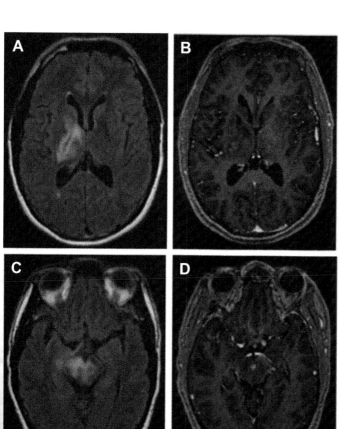

Fig. 10. A 47-year-old man with neuro-Behçet disease with recurrent oral ulcers, left arm and leg weakness, and diplopia with dysconjugate gaze. MR imaging shows FLAIR-hyperintense expansile lesions in the right lentiform nucleus, thalamus, internal capsule, mesial temporal lobe, and midbrain (A, C) with associated patchy enhancement (B, D).

gray and white matter and cortical lesions can occur (**Fig. 11**).[56] Hemorrhage is commonly parenchymal, unlike the convexity subarachnoid hemorrhage in RCVS.[32,36,56] Parenchymal or leptomeningeal enhancement can be seen, and occasionally the lesions are tumor-like.[16,36] Diagnostic criteria formulated by Hajj-Ali and colleagues[59] include (1) presence of an unexplained, acquired neurologic deficit after an extensive workup, (2) presence of an inflammatory arteritic process shown by pathology or angiography, and (3) absence of other systemic vasculitis. Biopsy remains the diagnostic gold standard but only yields up to a 61% positive rate because of sampling error.[56,57,60]

Vasculitis associated with systemic disease

Lupus vasculitis Systemic lupus erythematosus is an autoimmune disease with a wide range of clinical presentations, affecting women more than men. Patients with CNS involvement usually present with neuropsychiatric symptoms. CNS imaging shows infarctions of varied distribution and sizes, basal ganglia lesions, white matter T2/FLAIR hyperintensities, and vessel stenoses.[61–64] Lupus patients with positive antiphospholipid antibodies have an increased risk of thromboembolic phenomena such as infarctions and dural venous sinus thrombosis.[63,64] Cerebral atrophy, edema, hemorrhage, and intracranial calcifications can be seen.[61,64] VWI shows increased vessel wall lesions and infarct burden in lupus subjects compared with nonlupus subjects, even with normal-appearing vessels on MRA.[62]

Sarcoid vasculitis Sarcoidosis is an idiopathic inflammatory disease characterized by noncaseating granulomas, most commonly involving lungs, skin, and lymph nodes. CNS vessel imaging findings occur in up to 10% of patients, but pathologic involvement is much higher, with autopsy studies showing preferential involvement of small perforator branches within the Virchow-Robin spaces.[65–67] MRA and CTA usually do not have high enough resolution to detect abnormalities in

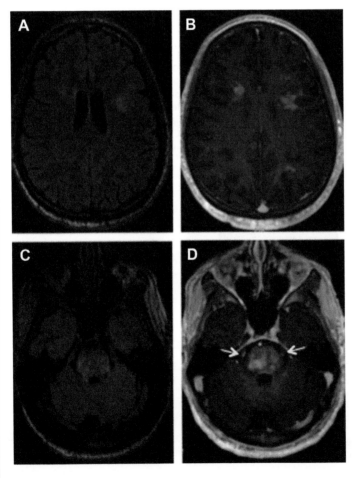

Fig. 11. A 28-year-old man with biopsy-proven primary angiitis of the CNS with facial numbness and pseudobulbar symptoms. MR imaging shows scattered FLAIR-hyperintense, enhancing frontal and parietal juxtacortical (*A, B*) and brainstem and left cerebellar (*C, D*) lesions. There is also enhancement of the cisternal segments of the trigeminal nerves (*arrows*).

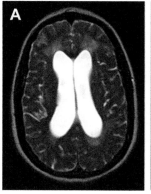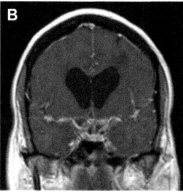

Fig. 12. A patient with neurosarcoidosis, hydrocephalus with T2-hyperintense transependymal edema (*A*), and basilar leptomeningeal enhancement (*B*).

the involved vessels.[66] The nonvascular CNS findings include leptomeningeal enhancement, especially of the basilar cisterns, nonenhancing periventricular white matter lesions, enhancing nodular or mass-like parenchymal lesions, cranial nerve enhancement, hydrocephalus, hypothalamic-pituitary axis enhancement and edema, enhancing dural lesions, spinal involvement, and lytic osseous lesions (**Fig. 12**).[67] Infarctions and hemorrhage are rare but may be the first presentation of neurosarcoidosis.[65,66]

Vasculitis associated with probable cause
This classification encompasses a heterogeneous group of vasculitides that result from specific causes (**Table 3**).

Table 3
Vasculitis associated with probable cause

Category	Cause
Infection	Varicella zoster virus/herpes simplex virus/cytomegalovirus
	HIV
	Hepatitis B virus
	Hepatitis C virus
	Tuberculosis
	Syphilis
Drugs	Hydralazine
	Cocaine
	Levamisole
	Minocycline
	Allopurinol
	Penicillamine
	Sulfasalazine
Neoplasm	Clonal B cell lymphoproliferative disorders
	Myelodysplastic syndrome
Other	Radiation

Infection Infectious CNS vasculitis may be from viral, bacterial, fungal, or parasitic causes. Common presentations include headaches, seizures, fevers, encephalopathy, stroke, and meningitis. Treatment varies by the infecting agent. On imaging, infected and inflamed intracranial vessels may show vascular remodeling, segmental narrowing, occlusion, and mycotic aneurysms. VWI can show wall thickening and transmural and periadventitial enhancement (**Fig. 13**). Serial vessel imaging may be helpful for monitoring treatment response. Other imaging findings include basilar meningeal enhancement (tuberculosis and bacterial infections), infarctions, and hemorrhage. Varicella zoster virus, one of the more common infectious vasculopathies, results in ischemic lesions, particularly of the deep gray and white matter and at gray-white matter junctions.[68]

Drugs Drug-induced CNS vasculitis has been associated with sympathomimetics, such as amphetamines, cocaine, and ephedrine.[69] Common clinical presentations include headaches, transient ischemic attacks, and stroke. It is noteworthy that drug-induced cerebral vasospasm is now considered part of the RCVS spectrum and can mimic the angiographic appearance of CNS vasculitis, which is much rarer.[58] Imaging findings include stenosis and occlusion, infarctions, and intraparenchymal hemorrhage. Histologically confirmed cases of angiitis are thought to have evolved from perivascular changes and vasculitis related to chronic vasoconstriction. Treatment is primarily aimed at removing the inciting agent.

Miscellaneous

Cerebral amyloid angiopathy
Cerebral amyloid angiopathy (CAA) comprises a spectrum of noninflammatory and inflammatory vasculopathies characterized by deposition of

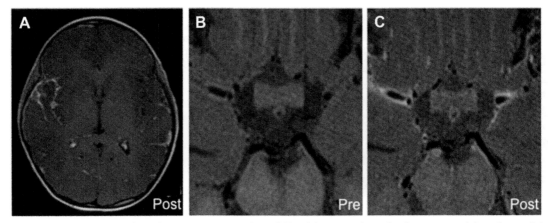

Fig. 13. A patient with tuberculous meningitis with multifocal leptomeningeal enhancement (*A*) and vasculitis with near circumferential wall enhancement of the bilateral proximal M1 middle cerebral arteries (*B, C*).

amyloid-β in vessel walls. CAA is most commonly a sporadic disease of the elderly, although a hereditary type presents at a younger age.[70] CAA typically presents with dementia or focal neurologic deficits and accounts for 5% to 20% of nontraumatic intracerebral hemorrhage in the elderly.[70,71] A diagnosis of probable CAA can be made with the modified Boston Criteria if (1) MR imaging or CT demonstrates multiple hemorrhages restricted to lobar, cortical, or cortical-subcortical regions (cerebellar hemorrhage allowed) or single lobar, cortical, or cortical-subcortical hemorrhage and superficial siderosis (focal or disseminated), (2) patient's age 55 years or older, and (3) there is no other hemorrhage cause.[72] SWI detects siderosis and microbleeds, which tend to be in a cortical-subcortical distribution with sparing of the basal ganglia, thalami, and brainstem (in contrast to hypertensive microbleeds).[71]

Inflammatory CAA (I-CAA) and amyloid-β–related angiitis (ABRA) are subtypes of CAA with similar features. I-CAA presents with perivascular inflammation without an angiodestructive component and is associated with the apoE ε4/ε4 genotype, while ABRA is a vasculitis with angiodestructive, often granulomatous, vessel wall inflammation and meningeal lymphocytosis.[73,74] The clinical presentation of I-CAA and ABRA are nonspecific, including altered mental status, headache, seizure, focal neurologic deficit, or hallucinations.[74,75] In contrast to noninflammatory CAA, MR imaging in I-CAA and ABRA shows asymmetric T2-hyperintense edema in a lobar, cortical, or subcortical distribution, as well as microbleeds and leptomeningeal enhancement concentrated in the areas of edema (**Fig. 14**).[71,73,75] It is important to recognize I-CAA and ABRA because they respond to immunosuppressants, unlike noninflammatory CAA.

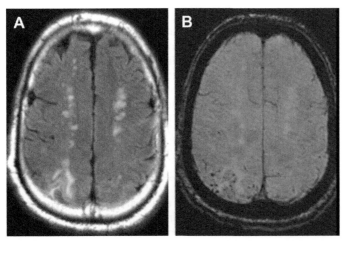

Fig. 14. A 70-year-old man with inflammatory cerebral amyloid angiopathy or amyloid-β–related angiitis with rapidly progressive dementia and psychosis. MR imaging shows hyperintense subcortical and cortical edema on FLAIR (*A*) and microhemorrhages on GRE (*B*) in the right parietal lobe.

SUMMARY

CNS vasculopathies are a diverse group of disorders with heterogeneous, and sometimes overlapping, clinical and imaging features. Identifying salient imaging features can help narrow differential diagnoses and guide appropriate treatment.

REFERENCES

1. Khosla A, Andring B, Atchie B, et al. Systemic vasculopathies: imaging and management. Radiol Clin North Am 2016;54(3):613–28.
2. Razek AAKA, Alvarez H, Bagg S, et al. Imaging spectrum of CNS vasculitis. Radiographics 2014; 34(4):873–94.
3. Jennette JC, Falk RJ, Bacon PA, et al. 2012 revised International Chapel Hill Consensus Conference Nomenclature of Vasculitides. Arthritis Rheum 2013;65(1):1–11.
4. Patel SG, Collie DA, Wardlaw JM, et al. Outcome, observer reliability, and patient preferences if CTA, MRA, or Doppler ultrasound were used, individually or together, instead of digital subtraction angiography before carotid endarterectomy. J Neurol Neurosurg Psychiatry 2002;73(1):21–8.
5. Czihal M, Lottspeich C, Hoffmann U. Ultrasound imaging in the diagnosis of large vessel vasculitis. Vasa 2017;46(4):241–53.
6. de Boysson H, Boulouis G, Parienti JJ, et al. Concordance of time-of-flight MRA and digital subtraction angiography in adult primary central nervous system vasculitis. AJNR Am J Neuroradiol 2017; 38(10):1917–22.
7. Heit JJ, Pastena GT, Nogueira RG, et al. Cerebral angiography for evaluation of patients with CT angiogram-negative subarachnoid hemorrhage: an 11-year experience. AJNR Am J Neuroradiol 2016; 37(2):297–304.
8. Obusez EC, Hui F, Hajj-ali RA, et al. High-resolution MRI vessel wall imaging: spatial and temporal patterns of reversible cerebral vasoconstriction syndrome and central nervous system vasculitis. AJNR Am J Neuroradiol 2014;35(8):1527–32.
9. Zeiler SR, Qiao Y, Pardo CA, et al. Vessel wall MRI for targeting biopsies of intracranial vasculitis. AJNR Am J Neuroradiol 2018;39(11):2034–6.
10. Mandell DM, Mossa-Basha M, Qiao Y, et al. Intracranial vessel wall MRI: principles and expert consensus recommendations of the American Society of Neuroradiology. AJNR Am J Neuroradiol 2017; 38(2):218–29.
11. Choi JC. Cerebral autosomal dominant arteriopathy with subcortical infarcts and leukoencephalopathy: a genetic cause of cerebral small vessel disease. J Clin Neurol 2010;6(1):1–9.
12. Dichgans M, Holtmannspötter M, Herzog J, et al. Cerebral microbleeds in CADASIL. Stroke 2002; 33(1):67–71.
13. Lee JS, Kang CH, Park SQ, et al. Clinical significance of cerebral microbleeds locations in CADASIL with R544C NOTCH3 mutation. PLoS One 2015;10(2):e0118163.
14. Susac JO, Murtagh FR, Egan RA, et al. MRI findings in Susac's syndrome. Neurology 2003;61(12):1783–7.
15. Buzzard KA, Reddel SW, Yiannikas C, et al. Distinguishing Susac's syndrome from multiple sclerosis. J Neurol 2015;(7):1613.
16. Garg A. Vascular brain pathologies. Neuroimaging Clin N Am 2011;21:897–926.
17. Mugikura S, Higano S, Shirane R, et al. Posterior circulation and high prevalence of ischemic stroke among young pediatric patients with moyamoya disease: evidence of angiography-based differences by age at diagnosis. AJNR Am J Neuroradiol 2011; 32(1):192–8.
18. Maeda M, Tsuchida C. "Ivy Sign" on fluid-attenuated inversion-recovery images in childhood moyamoya disease. AJNR Am J Neuroradiol 1999;20(10): 1836–8.
19. Lee S, Yun TJ, Yoo R-E, et al. Monitoring cerebral perfusion changes after revascularization in patients with moyamoya disease by using arterial spin-labeling MR imaging. Radiology 2018;288(2): 565–72.
20. Kuroda S, Kashiwazaki D, Ishikawa T, et al. Incidence, locations, and longitudinal course of silent microbleeds in moyamoya disease: a prospective T2*-weighted MRI study. Stroke 2013;44(2):516–8.
21. Yeon JY, Kim JS, Hong SC. Incidental major artery aneurysms in patients with non-hemorrhagic moyamoya disease. Acta Neurochir (Wien) 2011;153(6): 1263–70.
22. Olin JW, Gornik HL, Bacharach JM, et al. Fibromuscular dysplasia: state of the science and critical unanswered questions: a scientific statement from the American Heart Association. Circulation 2014; 129(9):1048–78.
23. O'Connor SC, Gornik HL. Recent developments in the understanding and management of fibromuscular dysplasia. J Am Heart Assoc 2014;3(6):e001259.
24. Olin JW, Froehlich J, Gu X, et al. The United States Registry for Fibromuscular Dysplasia: results in the first 447 patients. Circulation 2012;125(25):3182–90.
25. Zhang AJ, Dhruv P, Choi P, et al. A systematic literature review of patients with carotid web and acute ischemic stroke. Stroke 2018;12:2872.
26. Choi PM, Singh D, Trivedi A, et al. Carotid webs and recurrent ischemic strokes in the era of CT angiography. AJNR Am J Neuroradiol 2015;36(11):2134–9.
27. Kim ST, Brinjikji W, Lanzino G, et al. Neurovascular manifestations of connective-tissue diseases: a review. Interv Neuroradiol 2016;22(6):624–37.

28. Ha HI, Seo JB, Lee SH, et al. Imaging of Marfan syndrome: multisystemic manifestations. Radiographics 2007;27(4):989–1004.

29. Malfait F, Francomano C, Byers P, et al. The 2017 international classification of the Ehlers-Danlos syndromes. Am J Med Genet C Semin Med Genet 2017;175(1):8–26.

30. Loeys BL, Schwarze U, Holm T, et al. Aneurysm syndromes caused by mutations in the TGF-β receptor. N Engl J Med 2006;355(8):788–98.

31. Chu LC, Johnson PT, Dietz HC, et al. CT angiographic evaluation of genetic vascular disease: role in detection, staging, and management of complex vascular pathologic conditions. AJR Am J Roentgenol 2014;202(5):1120–9.

32. Singhal AB, Topcuoglu MA, Fok JW, et al. Reversible cerebral vasoconstriction syndromes and primary angiitis of the central nervous system: clinical, imaging, and angiographic comparison. Ann Neurol 2016;79(6):882–94.

33. Calabrese LH, Dodick DW, Schwedt TJ, et al. Narrative review: reversible cerebral vasoconstriction syndromes. Ann Intern Med 2007;146(1):34–44.

34. Miller TR, Shivashankar R, Mossa-Basha M, et al. Reversible cerebral vasoconstriction syndrome, part 1: epidemiology, pathogenesis, and clinical course. AJNR Am J Neuroradiol 2015;36(8):1392–9.

35. Ducros A. Reversible cerebral vasoconstriction syndrome. Lancet Neurol 2012;11(10):906–17.

36. de Boysson H, Parienti JJ, Mawet J, et al. Primary angiitis of the CNS and reversible cerebral vasoconstriction syndrome: a comparative study. Neurology 2018;91(16):e1468–78.

37. Miller TR, Shivashankar R, Mossa-Basha M, et al. Reversible cerebral vasoconstriction syndrome, part 2: diagnostic work-up, imaging evaluation, and differential diagnosis. AJNR Am J Neuroradiol 2015;36(9):1580–8.

38. de Souza AW, de Carvalho JF. Diagnostic and classification criteria of Takayasu arteritis. J Autoimmun 2014;48-49:79–83.

39. Gotway MB, Araoz PA, Macedo TA, et al. Imaging findings in Takayasu's arteritis. AJR Am J Roentgenol 2005;184(6):1945–50.

40. Pipitone N, Versari A, Salvarani C. Role of imaging studies in the diagnosis and follow-up of large-vessel vasculitis: an update. Rheumatology 2008; 47(4):403–8.

41. Barra L, Kanji T, Malette J, et al. Imaging modalities for the diagnosis and disease activity assessment of Takayasu's arteritis: a systematic review and meta-analysis. Autoimmun Rev 2018;17(2):175–87.

42. Choe YH, Han B-K, Koh E-M, et al. Takayasu's arteritis. AJR Am J Roentgenology 2000;175(2):505–11.

43. Slart RHJA, Slart RHJA, Glaudemans AWJM, et al. FDG-PET/CT(A) imaging in large vessel vasculitis and polymyalgia rheumatica: joint procedural recommendation of the EANM, SNMMI, and the PET Interest Group (PIG), and endorsed by the ASNC. Eur J Nucl Med Mol Imaging 2018;45(7): 1250–69.

44. Schmidt WA. Role of ultrasound in the understanding and management of vasculitis. Ther Adv Musculoskelet Dis 2014;6(2):39–47.

45. Klink T, Geiger J, Both M, et al. Giant cell arteritis: diagnostic accuracy of MR imaging of superficial cranial arteries in initial diagnosis—results from a multicenter trial. Radiology 2014;273(3):844–52.

46. Provenzale JM, Allen NB. Neuroradiologic findings in polyarteritis nodosa. AJNR Am J Neuroradiol 1996;17(6):1119–26.

47. Diagnostic guidelines for Kawasaki disease. Circulation 2001;103(2):335–6.

48. Okanishi T, Enoki H. Transient subcortical high-signal lesions in Kawasaki syndrome. Pediatr Neurol 2012;47(4):295–8.

49. De Luna G, Terrier B, Kaminsky P, et al. Central nervous system involvement of granulomatosis with polyangiitis: clinical-radiological presentation distinguishes different outcomes. Rheumatology 2015; 54(3):424–32.

50. Graf J. Central nervous system disease in antineutrophil cytoplasmic antibodies-associated vasculitis. Rheum Dis Clin North Am 2017;43(4):573–8.

51. Retamozo S, Díaz-Lagares C, Bosch X, et al. Life-threatening cryoglobulinemic patients with hepatitis C: clinical description and outcome of 279 patients. Medicine 2013;92(5):273–84.

52. Berube MD, Blais N, Lanthier S. Neurologic manifestations of Henoch-Schonlein purpura. Handb Clin Neurol 2014;120:1101–11.

53. Chae EJ, Do K-H, Seo JB, et al. Radiologic and clinical findings of Behçet disease: comprehensive review of multisystemic involvement. Radiographics 2008;28(5):e31.

54. Kalra S, Silman A, Akman-Demir G, et al. Diagnosis and management of Neuro-Behçet's disease: international consensus recommendations. J Neurol 2014;261(9):1662–76.

55. Matsuo K, Yamada K, Nakajima K, et al. Neuro-Behçet disease mimicking brain tumor. AJNR Am J Neuroradiol 2005;26(3):650–3.

56. Birnbaum J, Hellmann DB. Primary angiitis of the central nervous system. Arch Neurol 2009;66(6):704–9.

57. Alba MA, Espígol-Frigolé G, Prieto-González S, et al. Central nervous system vasculitis: still more questions than answers. Curr Neuropharmacol 2011; 9(3):437–48.

58. Salvarani C, Brown RD Jr, Hunder GG. Adult primary central nervous system vasculitis. Lancet 2012; 380(9843):767–77.

59. Hajj-Ali RA, Singhal AB, Benseler S, et al. Primary angiitis of the CNS. Lancet Neurol 2011;10(6): 561–72.

60. de Boysson H, Zuber M, Naggara O, et al. Primary angiitis of the central nervous system: description of the first fifty-two adults enrolled in the French cohort of patients with primary vasculitis of the central nervous system. Arthritis Rheumatol (Hoboken, NJ) 2014;66(5):1315–26.

61. Sibbitt WL Jr, Brooks WM, Kornfeld M, et al. Magnetic resonance imaging and brain histopathology in neuropsychiatric systemic lupus erythematosus. Semin Arthritis Rheum 2010;40(1):32–52.

62. Ide S, Kakeda S, Miyata M, et al. Intracranial vessel wall lesions in patients with systematic lupus erythematosus. J Magn Reson Imaging 2018;48(5): 1237–46.

63. Kaichi Y, Kakeda S, Moriya J, et al. Brain MR findings in patients with systemic lupus erythematosus with and without antiphospholipid antibody syndrome. AJNR Am J Neuroradiol 2014;35(1): 100–5.

64. Goh YP, Naidoo P, Ngian GS. Imaging of systemic lupus erythematosus. Part I: CNS, cardiovascular, and thoracic manifestations. Clin Radiol 2013; 68(2):181–91.

65. Bathla G, Watal P, Gupta S, et al. Cerebrovascular manifestations of neurosarcoidosis: an underrecognized aspect of the imaging spectrum. AJNR Am J Neuroradiol 2018;39(7):1194–200.

66. Jachiet V, Lhote R, Rufat P, et al. Clinical, imaging, and histological presentations and outcomes of stroke related to sarcoidosis. J Neurol 2018; 265(10):2333–41.

67. Smith JK, Matheus MG, Castillo M. Imaging manifestations of neurosarcoidosis. AJR Am J Roentgenology 2004;182(2):289–95.

68. Gilden D, Cohrs RJ, Mahalingam R, et al. Varicella zoster virus vasculopathies: diverse clinical manifestations, laboratory features, pathogenesis, and treatment. Lancet Neurol 2009;8(8):731–40.

69. Hogan JJ, Markowitz GS, Radhakrishnan J. Drug-induced glomerular disease: immune-mediated injury. Clin J Am Soc Nephrol 2015;10(7):1300–10.

70. Biffi A, Greenberg SM. Cerebral amyloid angiopathy: a systematic review. J Clin Neurol 2011;7(1): 1–9.

71. Miller-Thomas MM, Sipe AL, Benzinger TLS, et al. Multimodality review of amyloid-related diseases of the central nervous system. Radiographics 2016; 36(4):1147–63.

72. Greenberg SM, Charidimou A. Diagnosis of cerebral amyloid angiopathy. Stroke 2018;49(2):491–7.

73. Moussaddy A, Levy A, Strbian D, et al. Inflammatory cerebral amyloid angiopathy, amyloid-beta-related angiitis, and primary angiitis of the central nervous system: similarities and differences. Stroke 2015; 46(9):e210–3.

74. Scolding NJ, Joseph F, Kirby PA, et al. Abeta-related angiitis: primary angiitis of the central nervous system associated with cerebral amyloid angiopathy. Brain 2005;128(Pt 3):500–15.

75. Auriel E, Charidimou A, Gurol ME, et al. Validation of clinicoradiological criteria for the diagnosis of cerebral amyloid angiopathy-related inflammation. JAMA Neurol 2016;73(2):197–202.

Posterior Reversible Encephalopathy Syndrome and Reversible Cerebral Vasoconstriction Syndrome
Distinct Clinical Entities with Overlapping Pathophysiology

Alex Levitt, MD[a],*, Richard Zampolin, MD[b], Judah Burns, MD[b], Jacqueline A. Bello, MD[b], Shira E. Slasky, MD[b]

KEYWORDS

- Reversible cerebral vasoconstriction • Posterior reversible encephalopathy • Seizure • Brain

KEY POINTS

- Patients with posterior reversible encephalopathy syndrome (PRES) typically present with seizures and almost always show vasogenic edema involving the middle cerebral artery-posterior cerebral artery border zone in the parietal and occipital lobes.
- PRES has been associated with a variety of conditions known to cause endothelial damage: eclampsia, posttransplant immunosuppression, cancer chemotherapy, septic shock, and autoimmune disease.
- Reversible cerebral vasoconstriction syndrome (RCVS) is a clinical and radiographic syndrome in which patients present with thunderclap headache (a severe, throbbing headache that reaches peak intensity within 60 seconds of onset) and reversible cerebral artery vasoconstriction.
- RCVS is associated with vasoactive medications and/or the postpartum state in most cases. RCVS is an underdiagnosed entity. If recognized appropriately, unnecessary treatment may be avoided.
- PRES and RCVS often coexist and there is overlap among the disease entities associated with them. This finding suggests a common underlying pathophysiology.

INTRODUCTION

Posterior reversible encephalopathy syndrome (PRES) presents as a typical pattern of vasogenic edema, initially described in the setting of severe hypertension, eclampsia, and cyclosporine therapy after transplant, but has since been recognized in the setting of many additional systemic disorders.[1] Although the pattern of edema in PRES tends to be extensive, it almost always involves the middle cerebral artery (MCA)–posterior cerebral artery (PCA) arterial border zone of the occipital and parietal lobes. Patients with PRES typically present with generalized seizures, although acute headache and altered mental status are other common presentations.[2,3] The total incidence of PRES globally is unknown, although it has been reported in 3% to 16% of patients

Disclosure: None of the authors have any commercial or financial conflicts of interest related to this article.
[a] Jacobi Medical Center, Albert Einstein College of Medicine, 1400 Pelham Pkwy S, Bronx, NY 10461, USA;
[b] Montefiore Medical Center, 111 East 210th Street, Bronx, NY 10467, USA
* Corresponding author.
E-mail address: levitta@nychhc.org

Radiol Clin N Am 57 (2019) 1133–1146
https://doi.org/10.1016/j.rcl.2019.07.001

undergoing cyclosporine therapy after allogenic bone marrow transplant.[4] Most cases of PRES occur in young to middle-aged adults, although it has been reported at all ages. PRES is more common in women, which may reflect the epidemiology of the associated systemic disorders.[1] Management of PRES includes antiepileptic medication and treating the underlying cause. There is no evidence for use of glucocorticoids to treat the vasogenic edema.[5]

Reversible cerebral vasoconstriction syndrome (RCVS) is a clinical and radiographic syndrome in which patients present with thunderclap headache (a severe, throbbing headache that reaches peak intensity within 60 seconds of onset) and reversible cerebral artery vasoconstriction.[6] The term RCVS was proposed by Calabrese and colleagues[7] in 2007 as a way to recognize the similarities among entities with reversible vasoconstriction, such as postpartum angiopathy, migrainous vasospasm, primary thunderclap headache, drug-induced angiopathy, and Call-Fleming syndrome, initially considered to be unique clinical syndromes. Diagnostic criteria were proposed to emphasize the acute and severe nature of the headache, and the reversible clinical and angiographic findings, as well as to exclude alternative diagnoses such as aneurysmal subarachnoid hemorrhage (Box 1).[7] The incidence of RCVS is uncertain, but it does not seem to be rare based on the numbers of patients reported in prospective and retrospective studies.[8] Most cases of RCVS occur in young to middle-aged women.[8] Treatment of RCVS includes blood pressure control, seizure prophylaxis, analgesics to relieve symptoms, and withdrawal of any suspected triggers. Calcium channel blockers, via oral and intra-arterial routes, have been shown to provide symptom relief. Intra-arterial vasodilators and balloon angioplasty may improve vasoconstriction; however, recurrence has been reported.[6]

PRES is considered a distinct diagnostic entity but has overlapping features with RCVS. PRES-like reversible cerebral edema is encountered in between 9% and 38% of patients with RCVS, whereas most patients with PRES show some element of cerebral arterial vasoconstriction when conventional angiography is performed.[9,10] When PRES-like features are encountered in cases of RCVS, the anatomic distribution of cerebral edema is similar to PRES encountered in other settings.[11] RCVS also shows similar clinical features to PRES, including acute headache, confusion, and seizures.[8] Toxemia of pregnancy has been associated with PRES and mirrors the association of RCVS with the postpartum state.[12–14] Given the significant overlap between the two entities, it is likely that RCVS and PRES share a common pathophysiology.[6]

PATHOPHYSIOLOGIC MECHANISMS AND ASSOCIATED CONDITIONS
Posterior Reversible Encephalopathy Syndrome

Endothelial damage is common to the pathophysiology of almost all of the conditions associated with PRES: eclampsia, posttransplant immunosuppression, cancer chemotherapy, septic shock, and autoimmune disease (Box 2).[10,15–17] Diffuse endothelial injury results in decreased production of endothelium-derived vasorelaxants and systemic vasoconstriction.[18,19] One proposed mechanism for PRES is hypoperfusion in the setting of endothelial damage and systemic vasoconstriction.[2] Hypertension may occur, designed to increase perfusion and reverse brain hypoxemia. This theory helps to explain the arterial border-zone distribution of PRES.

An alternative mechanism for PRES is hypertension with failed autoregulation, causing capillary injury and hyperperfusion.[2] This theory suggests that as blood pressure exceeds the limits of cerebral autoregulation, passive arteriolar dilatation leads to capillary injury, resulting in vessel injury and vasogenic edema. Sparse sympathetic innervation of the posterior circulation results in less protective vasoconstriction and can be invoked to explain the posterior predominance of PRES.[20]

Arguing against a causative role for hypertension in PRES is the absence of hypertension in 20% to 30% of PRES cases. In addition,

---

Box 1
Reversible cerebral vasoconstriction syndrome diagnostic criteria: The International Classification of Headache Disorders, Third Edition

Severe acute headaches with or without seizures or neurologic deficits

Self-limited, monophasic course, with resolution of symptoms within 3 months of onset

Headache not accounted for by another diagnosis, especially aneurysmal subarachnoid hemorrhage

Multifocal cerebral artery vasoconstriction

Reversibility of angiographic findings within 3 months of onset

Data from International Headache Society. International Classification of Headache Disorders, Third Edition (ICHD-3). International Headache Society; 2013. Available at: https://ichd-3.org/.

Box 2
Risk factors associated with posterior reversible encephalopathy syndrome

Hypertension

Preeclampsia/eclampsia (toxemia of pregnancy)

Posttransplant

Immunosuppression

Infection, sepsis, and shock

Autoimmune disease

- Systemic sclerosis (scleroderma)
- Granulomatosis with polyangiitis (Wegener)
- Polyarteritis nodosa
- Systemic lupus erythematosus

Cancer chemotherapy

Metabolic disorders

- Hypercalcemia
- Hypomagnesemia

Other

- Intravenous immunoglobulin
- Guillain-Barré syndrome
- Ephedra overdose
- Dialysis/erythropoietin
- Triple-H therapy
- Tumor lysis syndrome

hypertension in most patients with PRES does not exceed cerebral autoregulatory limits.[2,21] Some studies have failed to find a correlation between degree of hypertension and severity of PRES edema,[3,16] whereas others have found inverse correlations,[9,22] unexpected findings if considering failed autoregulation as the primary mechanism behind PRES. For these reasons, endothelial damage with systemic vasoconstriction and brain hypoperfusion is more central to the cause of PRES than hypertension. However, it is possible that hypertension in conjunction with endothelial damage may make some contribution to the vasogenic edema seen in PRES and help to explain its posterior predominance.

Hypercalcemia is associated with PRES independent of endothelial damage and may act on the arterial media to impair vasodilatation.[23–25] Magnesium is a competitive antagonist to calcium, and hypomagnesemia has also been associated with PRES. A review by Chardain and colleagues[26] found acute hypomagnesemia in 19 consecutive patients with PRES.

A proposed mechanism for the blood-brain barrier breakdown seen in PRES is tissue hypoxia and vascular endothelial growth factor (VEGF) upregulation, stimulating angiogenesis and increasing endothelial permeability.[27] However, multiple cases of PRES have been reported in the setting of bevacizumab, a VEGF inhibitor.[28–30] Moreover, increased production of soluble fms-like tyrosine kinase 1 (sFLT1), a circulating antagonist to VEGF, has been documented in the placentas of preeclamptic women and is sufficient to induce hypertension and pathologic changes of preeclampsia in animal models.[31] These findings suggest that VEGF receptor antagonism could be a mechanism for PRES and that upregulation of VEGF may represent a secondary response to this.

Reversible Cerebral Vasoconstriction Syndrome

Most cases of RCVS are associated with vasoactive drugs (~50% of cases) or the postpartum state (~10% of cases) (Box 3). The association of RCVS with migraine headaches (20%–40% of cases) is likely caused by the vasoactive effects of many migraine medications. Many cases of RCVS also develop spontaneously, without a clear underlying cause.[6]

Endothelial vasoconstriction may be triggered directly by vasoactive substances. The mechanisms by which the postpartum state could cause RCVS are less clear. RCVS has been observed in nonpregnant patients with sudden decreases in the concentration of estrogens and progesterones, suggesting a hormonal contribution to RCVS pathogenesis.[8,32–34] RCVS has also been documented in the antepartum state in association with PRES, suggesting nonhormonal mechanisms are at play.[35] Although the label RCVS may not have been explicitly used, vasoconstriction characteristic of the syndrome has been documented in multiple cases of eclampsia, in both the antepartum and postpartum periods.[10,13,36]

Ducros and colleagues[37] proposed that the vasoconstriction observed in RCVS starts in small distal arteries and progresses centrally toward medium-sized and large arteries. This theory helps to account for observations of thunderclap headaches in the absence of vasoconstriction as well as the persistence of vasoconstriction after headache resolution. Vasoconstriction of small distal arteries undetectable on angiography may stimulate trigeminal leptomeningeal afferents to induce thunderclap headache. Headache resolution likely coincides with resolution of this peripheral vasoconstriction while it progresses centripetally to involve

> **Box 3**
> **Potential triggers of reversible cerebral vasoconstriction syndrome**
>
> Vasoactive medications
> - Sympathomimetic drugs
> - Bromocriptine
> - Ergotamine
> - Pseudoephedrine
> - Selective serotonin uptake inhibitors
> - Interferon
> - Triptans
> - Diet pills
> - Nonsteroidal antiinflammatory drugs
>
> Vasoactive recreational drugs
> - Alcohol
> - Amphetamines
> - Cannabis
> - Cocaine
> - Ecstasy
> - Nicotine
>
> Pregnancy and postpartum states[a]
>
> Blood products: transfusions, erythropoietin[a], intravenous immunoglobulin[a]
>
> Headache disorders: migraines
>
> Tumors: pheochromocytoma, paraganglioma
>
> Trauma
>
> Other
> - HELP –(hemolysis, elevated liver enzymes, low platelets) syndrome
> - Antiphospholipid antibody syndrome
> - Thrombotic thrombocytopenic purpura
>
> Carotid dissection, unruptured cerebral aneurysm
>
> Head and neck surgery
>
> [a] Also associated with PRES.

medium-sized and large arteries that then become evident on angiography.

IMAGING, PATHOLOGY, AND DIFFERENTIAL DIAGNOSIS
Posterior Reversible Encephalopathy Syndrome: Imaging and Pathology

The basic PRES pattern can be recognized by cortical and juxtacortical fluid-attenuated inversion recovery (FLAIR) hyperintensity primarily in the parietal and occipital cortex, although most cases show additional involvement of the frontal and temporal lobes. In addition to the dominant parietal-occipital pattern (MCA/PCA border zone), other patterns of edema have been described. These patterns include the holohemispheric pattern (anterior cerebral artery [ACA]/MCA/PCA border zones), superior frontal sulcus pattern (ACA/MCA border zones), as well as partial or asymmetric expression of these patterns (Fig. 1).[21]

Involvement of the deep white matter, basal ganglia, brainstem, and cerebellum (Fig. 2), as well as restricted diffusion, hemorrhage, and contrast enhancement (Fig. 3), have been reported in a minority of PRES cases.[3,21] If cerebellar or brainstem involvement are extensive, hydrocephalus or brainstem compression may occur.[38] Foci of restricted diffusion and hemorrhage imply irreversible parenchymal damage, often evolving to encephalomalacia.[21] Apparent diffusion coefficient values may be normal or even increased in infarcts secondary to intravoxel averaging of both cytotoxic and vasogenic edema in cortex affected by PRES.[39] Therefore increased signal on diffusion-weighted imaging (DWI) alone is an important finding, especially if the patient has a focal neurologic deficit.

Multiple case series document hypoperfusion in PRES on single-photon emission CT and magnetic resonance perfusion imaging, although typically more than a day after onset of the patient's symptoms.[40,41] There are several case reports of PRES with documented hyperperfusion, with imaging in these cases performed in the setting of acute hypertension or within a day of the patient's symptoms.[20] Understanding that vasogenic edema in PRES reduces local perfusion under any circumstance, it is important to consider the timing of perfusion data in these studies and interpret their results with caution.[42]

Most patients with PRES (85%) show some element of cerebral arterial vasoconstriction when conventional angiography is performed.[1,10] Autopsy studies in PRES show evidence of acute and chronic vessel injury with intimal thickening, segmental vessel narrowing, and organized thrombi.[1] Similarly, in an autopsy series of 19 patients with eclampsia, a condition closely associated with PRES, loss of endothelial-specific markers and expansion of perivascular Virchow-Robin spaces was noted, compatible with endothelial injury.[43,44] It is interesting that these findings of endothelial injury were not associated with larger arteries except in cases of parenchymal infarction. The investigators acknowledged that systemic

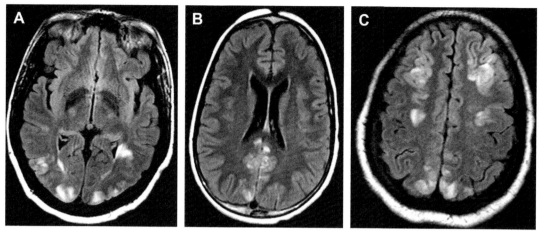

Fig. 1. Typical patterns of edema in PRES. Axial T2 FLAIR images show cortical edema in arterial border-zone distributions seen in PRES. (*A*) MCA-PCA, (*B*) ACA/PCA, (*C*) ACA/MCA.

endothelial injury may also be shown on histopathology in the setting of malignant hypertension.

Posterior Reversible Encephalopathy Syndrome: Differential Diagnosis

Hypoxic ischemic encephalopathy

Hypoxic ischemic encephalopathy (HIE) can lead to a pattern of edema similar to PRES (**Box 4, Fig. 4**). In the acute setting of HIE, the DWI signal abnormality tends to be more prominent than the accompanying abnormal FLAIR signal.[3] However, in the subacute period this finding is no longer reliable because the DWI signal abnormality fades, whereas the FLAIR signal abnormality persists.[45] A more reliable way to distinguish between these entities is involvement of the deep gray matter, which occurs in almost all cases of HIE but only a small minority of cases of PRES.[46,47]

Bilateral subacute posterior border-zone infarcts

Acute infarcts typically present with a unilateral distribution in an arterial vascular territory and cytotoxic pattern of edema. This pattern can be distinguished from PRES, which typically presents with a bilateral arterial border-zone distribution and a vasogenic pattern of edema. However, bilateral subacute posterior watershed infarcts may be difficult to distinguish from PRES, particularly because PRES may progress to irreversible injury.[48]

Postictal state

Reversible brain edema may also be seen in the postictal setting and resemble PRES.

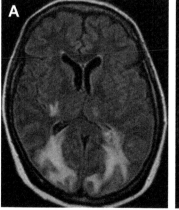
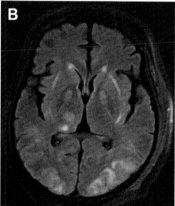
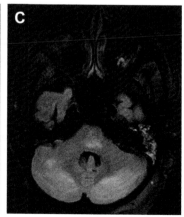

Fig. 2. Atypical distributions in PRES. Axial T2 FLAIR images show edema in the (*A*) deep white matter, (*B*) basal ganglia, (*C*) cerebellum and brainstem.

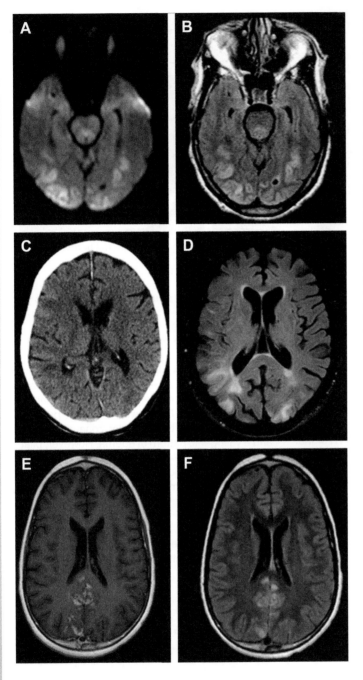

Fig. 3. Uncommon imaging findings in PRES. (A) Axial diffusion-weighted image shows cortical hyperintensity in the MCA-PCA border zones with corresponding hypointensity on apparent diffusion coefficient (not shown), compatible with restricted diffusion. (B) Axial T2 FLAIR image at the same level confirms typical imaging features of PRES. (C) Axial computed tomography (CT) image in a different patient shows right perisylvian subarachnoid hemorrhage. (D) Axial T2 FLAIR image at a similar level confirms typical imaging features of PRES. Note the corresponding right perisylvian sulcal hyperintensity compatible with subarachnoid hemorrhage. (E) Axial contrast-enhanced T1-weighted image in a different patient shows leptomeningeal enhancement in the region of the parieto-occipital sulcus and splenium of the corpus callosum. (F) Axial T2 FLAIR image at the same level confirms typical imaging features of PRES.

Seizures are the most common presenting symptom in PRES, which may confound these two entities. Hippocampal involvement and unilateral distribution suggest postictal changes rather than PRES because the hippocampus is not a classic watershed arterial vascular territory and PRES almost always has a bilateral distribution.[49] Unilateral distribution was characteristic of half of the peri-ictal patients described in a study by Cianfoni and colleagues[50] but only present in 2 out of 76 patients described in a PRES case series by McKinney and colleagues.[3] In addition, based on our clinical experience, postictal changes are typically centered in the cortex without significant subcortical white matter involvement. Splenial involvement is atypical for PRES but may be seen in the postictal setting.[46]

Box 4
Differential diagnosis of posterior reversible encephalopathy syndrome

HIE

Postictal state

Bilateral subacute posterior border-zone infarcts

Other causes of reversible vasogenic edema

- Hypertensive encephalopathy
- Acute toxic leukoencephalopathy

Other conditions with reversible vasogenic edema

Rare cases of reversible vasogenic edema sparing the supratentorial cortical watersheds with involvement of the brainstem and basal ganglia have been described in the setting of acute hypertensive crises.[3,51–53] Reversible vasogenic edema has also been reported following carotid endarterectomy involving the ipsilateral cerebral hemisphere.[54] Given the consistent association with blood pressures exceeding autoregulation, absence of conditions associated with systemic endothelial damage, and no documentation of cerebral vasoconstriction, it is unclear whether these entities represent PRES variants or distinct pathophysiologic entities.

Acute toxic leukoencephalopathy is characterized by acute neurologic deterioration with reversible vasogenic edema and restricted diffusion in the periventricular white matter. This entity occurs in the setting of many of the same medications and drugs associated with PRES; however, it should be easily distinguished by its predominant involvement of the periventricular white matter and lack of cortical involvement.[55]

Reversible Cerebral Vasoconstriction Syndrome: Imaging and Pathology

At initial clinical presentation, brain imaging of many patients with RCVS, including angiography, may appear unremarkable, highlighting the high degree of clinical suspicion necessary when patients present with thunderclap headaches.[56] A proposed imaging correlate for this angiographically occult peripheral arterial vasoconstriction is slow flow in leptomeningeal vessels, manifesting as increased T2 FLAIR signal, appearing tubular when the vessels are in plane and dotlike when out of plane.[56]

Noncisternal subarachnoid hemorrhage is the most common hemorrhagic complication of RCVS, occurring in approximately one-third of patients. Subarachnoid hemorrhage and PRES, occurring in a minority of RCVS cases, both typically present within the first week of clinical symptoms.[57,58] Ischemic strokes occur in a minority of patients, typically in a cortical arterial watershed distribution occurring more than 1 week after initial clinical onset.[8] The earlier onset of subarachnoid hemorrhage and PRES is hypothesized to reflect the sequela of smaller and more peripherally located artery vasoconstriction, whereas the later onset of positive angiographic studies and ischemic stroke is thought to reflect the sequela of larger and more centrally located artery vasoconstriction (**Figs. 5** and **6**).[8,56]

Angiography shows beaded arterial vasoconstriction that is out of proportion to the degree of subarachnoid hemorrhage, if present. A study of 77 patients with RCVS by Chen and colleagues[11] showed that peak arterial vasoconstriction occurs at approximately 16 days after symptom onset, around the same time as headache resolution. Sensitivity of indirect angiography is about 70% that of catheter angiography, which likely relates to the superior spatial resolution of conventional angiography in evaluating small distal cerebral arteries.[8,59] Intra-arterial administration of nimodipine has been proposed as a means of diagnosing RCVS by completely reversing vasoconstriction, distinguishing it from other entities such as primary angiitis of the central nervous system (PACNS), moyamoya, or arteriosclerotic disease, which show only partial improvement.[60] Transcranial Doppler has also been used to diagnose and monitor vasoconstriction in patients with RCVS.[8]

Brain biopsies in RCVS have shown normal arterial histology with the absence of vessel wall inflammation seen in vasculitis.[8]

Reversible Cerebral Vasoconstriction Syndrome: Differential Diagnosis

Aneurysmal subarachnoid hemorrhage

Headache caused by a sentinel hemorrhage from a brain aneurysm could be clinically indistinguishable from a thunderclap headache in the setting of RCVS, although their imaging features are different (**Box 5, Figs. 7** and **8**). Subarachnoid hemorrhage with basal cistern predominance, and subsequent vasospasm of long segments of the proximal arteries, is characteristic of aneurysmal subarachnoid hemorrhage. Focal subarachnoid hemorrhage along the cerebral convexities with a disproportionate beaded

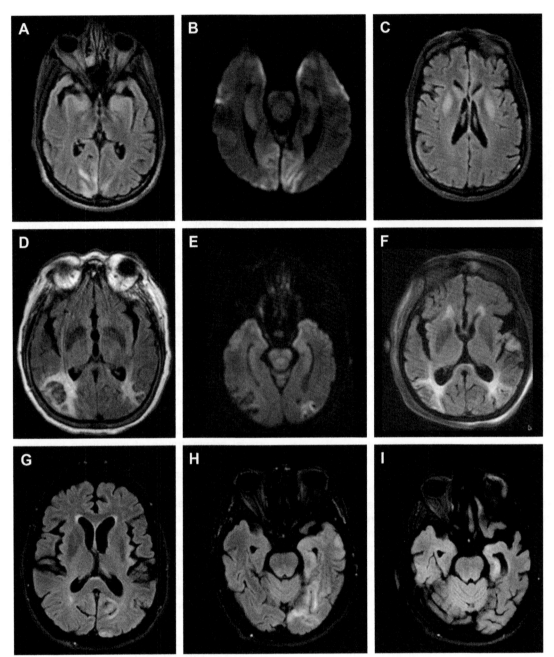

Fig. 4. Differential diagnosis of PRES. (*A–C*) HIE. (*A*) Axial T2 FLAIR image shows increased signal in the cortex and juxtacortical white matter of the medial occipital lobes, which may suggest PRES. (*B*) However, DWI in the same patient shows restricted diffusion in the medial occipital cortex. (*C*) Axial T2 FLAIR image in the same patient shows involvement the caudate nuclei and putamina. Although basal ganglia involvement and cortical restricted diffusion can be seen in a minority of PRES cases, they rarely are seen in combination. Moreover, the medial aspect of the occipital lobes is not a typical distribution for the cortical MCA/PCA border zone. (*D–F*) Acute and subacute posterior border-zone infarcts. (*D*) Axial T2 FLAIR image shows increased signal in the subcortical and periventricular white matter of the posterior temporal lobes, which might be mistaken for PRES. Note the concomitant presence of subcortical hypointense signal representing hemorrhage. (*E*) DWI shows restricted diffusion in the left posterior temporal lobe, compatible with acute infarct. Note the absence of restricted diffusion on the right, suggestive of subacute infarct. (*F*) Axial T2 FLAIR image obtained 11 months later shows encephalomalacia and gliosis in the posterior border zones, compatible with chronic infarcts. Although infarcts and hemorrhage can occur in a minority of PRES cases, the asymmetric restricted diffusion on presentation and evolution to encephalomalacia and gliosis make this scenario less likely. (*G–I*) Postictal state. (*G*) Axial T2 FLAIR image shows

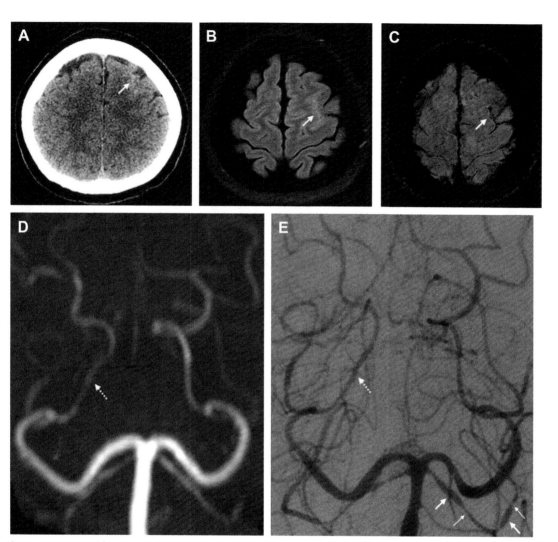

Fig. 5. A 47-year-old woman without a significant past medical history who presented with thunderclap head-aches. (*A*) Axial CT, (*B*) axial FLAIR, and (*C*) axial susceptibility-weighted images showing subtle subarachnoid hemorrhage within the left superior frontal sulcus (*arrows*). Note the linear susceptibility-related loss of signal across the entire left superior frontal sulcus in contrast with the dots and dashes seen on the contralateral side, representing leptomeningeal vessels. (*D*) Magnetic resonance angiography (MRA) showing asymmetric narrowing of the right medial occipital artery (*dotted arrow*). In retrospect, a thick-thin appearance (sausage-on-a-string appearance or beading) of the right superior cerebellar artery is present. (*E*) Digital subtraction angi-ography (DSA) showing multifocal alternating vascular stenoses and relative dilatations, as indicated by the white arrows, which highlight the left superior cerebellar artery. On close inspection, this pattern is seen throughout the imaged posterior circulation. In addition, note the partial resolution of this pattern by comparing the right medial occipital artery on the MRA with the DSA (*dotted arrow*) performed 3 days later. This finding provides evidence of partial reversibility.

increased signal in the left medial occipital cortex and subcortical white matter, which could resemble PRES. Note also the increased signal in the left posterior insula and left medial thalamus. (*H*) Axial T2 FLAIR image shows more extensive increased signal in the cortex and subcortical white matter along the left medial occipital and temporal lobes, including the hippocampus. (*I*) Axial T2 FLAIR image on follow-up shows residual increased signal in the left hippocampus. Although unilateral involvement of the occipital lobe can be seen in a minority of PRES cases, the involvement of the hippocampus and absence of contralateral involvement strongly suggests postictal changes rather than PRES.

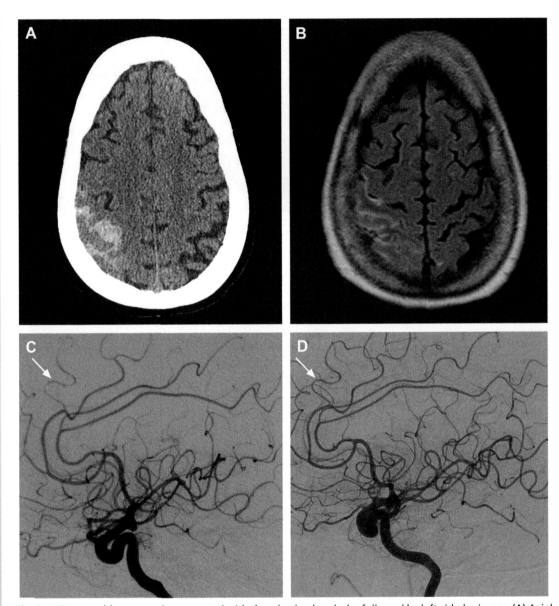

Fig. 6. A 71-year-old woman who presented with thunderclap headache followed by left-sided seizures. (A) Axial CT and (B) axial FLAIR images show right parietal subarachnoid hemorrhage. (C) DSA shows alternating stenoses and dilatations (*arrow*) of an anteromedial frontal branch off the callosomarginal artery. (D) Follow-up DSA 2 months later shows normal caliber of this vessel (*arrow*), with complete resolution.

peripheral vasoconstriction is characteristic of RCVS.[59] Although cisternal hemorrhage has been documented in a few cases of RCVS, this is the exception rather than the rule.[57]

Box 5
Differential diagnosis of reversible cerebral vasoconstriction syndrome

Aneurysmal subarachnoid hemorrhage

PACNS

Migraine headaches

Primary angiitis of the central nervous system

Differentiating RCVS from primary angiitis of the central nervous system (PACNS) is critical: giving patients with RCVS glucocorticoids has been associated with clinical worsening, whereas delaying immunosuppressive therapy in patients with PACNS is associated with a poor prognosis.[59,61] Large retrospective studies have shown that, in most cases, these entities can be distinguished based on clinical and imaging findings. Recurrent thunderclap headache or a single thunderclap headache in association with normal brain imaging, cortical-only infarction, or PRES occurs in

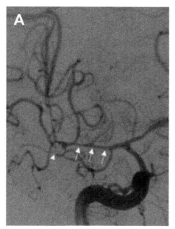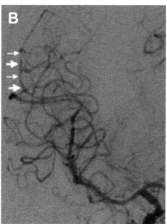

Fig. 7. RCVS differential diagnosis part 1. (*A*) DSA showing vasospasm (*arrows*) involving a long segment of the proximal right MCA. Note the right M2 bifurcation aneurysm coils (*arrowhead*) placed 1 week earlier at the site of aneurysmal subarachnoid hemorrhage. (*B*) DSA showing a thick-thin appearance (*thick and thin white arrows*) of a distal right MCA branch in the setting of RCVS.

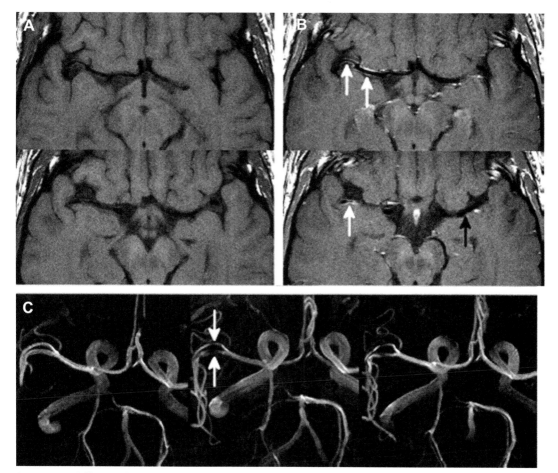

Fig. 8. RCVS differential diagnosis part 2. Central nervous system vasculitis. Axial T1-weighted vessel wall MR images before (*A*) and after (*B*) gadolinium at presentation show arterial wall thickening and enhancement (*arrows*). MR angiogram at the time of vessel wall imaging (*C, middle*) shows narrowing of the right MCA (*arrows*) compared with an MR angiogram obtained 2 months earlier (*C, left*). Follow-up angiogram 3 months after vessel wall MR imaging (*C, right*) shows persistent narrowing. RCVS would show absent/minimal vessel wall enhancement with resolution of the arterial narrowing over time. (*From* Mandell DM, Matouk CC, Farb RI, et al. Vessel wall MRI to differentiate between reversible cerebral vasoconstriction syndrome and central nervous system vasculitis: preliminary results. Stroke 2012;43:860-2. with permission.)

almost all RCVS cases but almost never in PACNS.[62,63] Deep brainstem infarcts and abnormal cerebrospinal fluid were seen in most PACNS cases and rarely in RCVS.[62,63] Given that angiography has limited sensitivity, the findings are nonspecific, and brain biopsy is diagnostic in less than half of cases, there may be a role for vessel wall imaging in ambiguous cases, which has shown promising results in multiple small studies.[64,65]

Recently, Rocha and colleagues[66] developed and validated the RCVS$_2$ score (based on the presence of thunderclap headache, the absence of intracranial carotid artery involvement, the presence of a vasoconstrictive trigger, patient's sex, and the presence of subarachnoid hemorrhage), to distinguish RCVS from other large-vessel/medium-vessel arteriopathies such as PACNS. The investigators found that the RCVS$_2$ score had a high sensitivity and specificity for the diagnosis and the exclusion of RCVS.[66]

Migraine
Patients with migraine with RCVS may initially complain of a worst-ever migraine attack; however, careful questioning can elicit a history of pain peaking within seconds, suggesting a diagnosis of RCVS.[8]

SUMMARY

PRES and RCVS represent distinct clinical entities but have overlapping pathophysiology related to endothelial damage and vasoconstriction. It is crucial to recognize the imaging manifestations of these two entities, to exclude alternative diagnoses, avoid inappropriate treatment, and provide the appropriate supportive therapy.

REFERENCES

1. Bartynski WS. Posterior reversible encephalopathy syndrome, part 1: fundamental imaging and clinical features. AJNR Am J Neuroradiol 2008;29: 1036–42.
2. Bartynski WS. Posterior reversible encephalopathy syndrome, part 2: controversies surrounding pathophysiology of vasogenic edema. AJNR Am J Neuroradiol 2008;29:1043–9.
3. McKinney AM, Short J, Truwit CL, et al. Posterior reversible encephalopathy syndrome: incidence of atypical regions of involvement and imaging findings. AJR Am J Roentgenol 2007;189:904–12.
4. Bartynski WS, Zeigler ZR, Shadduck RK, et al. Pretransplantation conditioning influence on the occurrence of cyclosporine or FK-506 neurotoxicity in allogeneic bone marrow transplantation. AJNR Am J Neuroradiol 2004;25:261–9.
5. Roth C, Ferbert A. The posterior reversible encephalopathy syndrome: what's certain, what's new? Pract Neurol 2011;11:136–44.
6. Miller TR, Shivashankar R, Mossa-Basha M, et al. Reversible cerebral vasoconstriction syndrome, part 1: epidemiology, pathogenesis, and clinical course. AJNR Am J Neuroradiol 2015;36:1392–9.
7. Calabrese LH, Dodick DW, Schwedt TJ, et al. Narrative review: reversible cerebral vasoconstriction syndromes. Ann Intern Med 2007;146:34–44.
8. Ducros A. Reversible cerebral vasoconstriction syndrome. Lancet Neurol 2012;11:906–17.
9. Bartynski WS, Boardman JF. Catheter angiography, MR angiography, and MR perfusion in posterior reversible encephalopathy syndrome. AJNR Am J Neuroradiol 2008;29:447–55.
10. Sengar AR, Gupta RK, Dhanuka AK, et al. MR imaging, MR angiography, and MR spectroscopy of the brain in eclampsia. AJNR Am J Neuroradiol 1997; 18:1485–90.
11. Chen SP, Fuh JL, Wang SJ, et al. Magnetic resonance angiography in reversible cerebral vasoconstriction syndromes. Ann Neurol 2010;67: 648–56.
12. Fugate JE, Wijdicks EF, Parisi JE, et al. Fulminant postpartum cerebral vasoconstriction syndrome. Arch Neurol 2012;69:111–7.
13. Singhal AB. Postpartum angiopathy with reversible posterior leukoencephalopathy. Arch Neurol 2004; 61:411–6.
14. Singhal AB, Bernstein RA. Postpartum angiopathy and other cerebral vasoconstriction syndromes. Neurocrit Care 2005;3:91–7.
15. Aird WC. The role of the endothelium in severe sepsis and multiple organ dysfunction syndrome. Blood 2003;101:3765–77.
16. Bartynski WS, Tan HP, Boardman JF, et al. Posterior reversible encephalopathy syndrome after solid organ transplantation. AJNR Am J Neuroradiol 2008; 29:924–30.
17. Gupta S, Kaplan MJ. Pathogenesis of systemic lupus erythematosus. In: Hochberg MC, Gravallese EM, Silman AJ, et al, editors. Rheumatology. 7th edition. Philadelphia: Elsevier; 2019. p. 1154–9.
18. Loscalzo J. Endothelial injury, vasoconstriction, and its prevention. Tex Heart Inst J 1995;22:180–4.
19. Sandoo A, van Zanten JJ, Metsios GS, et al. The endothelium and its role in regulating vascular tone. Open Cardiovasc Med J 2010;4:302–12.
20. Schwartz RB, Jones KM, Kalina P, et al. Hypertensive encephalopathy: findings on CT, MR imaging, and SPECT imaging in 14 cases. AJR Am J Roentgenol 1992;159:379–83.
21. Bartynski WS, Boardman JF. Distinct imaging patterns and lesion distribution in posterior reversible

encephalopathy syndrome. AJNR Am J Neuroradiol 2007;28:1320–7.

22. Bartynski WS, Boardman JF, Zeigler ZR, et al. Posterior reversible encephalopathy syndrome in infection, sepsis, and shock. AJNR Am J Neuroradiol 2006;27:2179–90.

23. Kaplan PW. Reversible hypercalcemic cerebral vasoconstriction with seizures and blindness: a paradigm for eclampsia? Clin Electroencephalogr 1998;29:120–3.

24. Kastrup O, Maschke M, Wanke I, et al. Posterior reversible encephalopathy syndrome due to severe hypercalcemia. J Neurol 2002;249:1563–6.

25. Neunteufl T, Katzenschlager R, Abela C, et al. Impairment of endothelium-independent vasodilation in patients with hypercalcemia. Cardiovasc Res 1998;40:396–401.

26. Chardain A, Mesnage V, Alamowitch S, et al. Posterior reversible encephalopathy syndrome (PRES) and hypomagnesemia: a frequent association? Revue Neurol (Paris) 2016;172:384–8.

27. Schoch HJ, Fischer S, Marti HH. Hypoxia-induced vascular endothelial growth factor expression causes vascular leakage in the brain. Brain 2002; 125:2549–57.

28. Cross SN, Ratner E, Rutherford TJ, et al. Bevacizumab-mediated interference with VEGF signaling is sufficient to induce a preeclampsia-like syndrome in nonpregnant women. Rev Obstet Gynecol 2012; 5:2–8.

29. Hamid M, Ghani A, Micaily I, et al. Posterior reversible encephalopathy syndrome (PRES) after bevacizumab therapy for metastatic colorectal cancer. J Community Hosp Intern Med Perspect 2018;8: 130–3.

30. Seet RC, Rabinstein AA. Clinical features and outcomes of posterior reversible encephalopathy syndrome following bevacizumab treatment. QJM 2012;105:69–75.

31. Harper LM, Tita A, Ananth Karumanchi S. Pregnancy-related hypertension. In: Robert Resnik CJL, Moore TR, Greene MF, et al, editors. Creasy and Resnik's maternal-fetal medicine: principles and practice E-book. Philadelphia: Elsevier; 2019. p. 810–38.

32. Freilinger T, Schmidt C, Duering M, et al. Reversible cerebral vasoconstriction syndrome associated with hormone therapy for intrauterine insemination. Cephalalgia 2010;30:1127–32.

33. Moussavi M, Korya D, Panezai S, et al. Reversible cerebral vasoconstriction syndrome in a 35-year-old woman following hysterectomy and bilateral salpingo-oophorectomy. J Neurointerv Surg 2012; 4:e35.

34. Soo Y, Singhal AB, Leung T, et al. Reversible cerebral vasoconstriction syndrome with posterior leucoencephalopathy after oral contraceptive pills. Cephalalgia 2010;30:42–5.

35. Tanaka K, Matsushima M, Matsuzawa Y, et al. Antepartum reversible cerebral vasoconstriction syndrome with pre-eclampsia and reversible posterior leukoencephalopathy. J Obstet Gynaecol Res 2015;41:1843–7.

36. Bartynski WS, Sanghvi A. Neuroimaging of delayed eclampsia. Report of 3 cases and review of the literature. J Comput Assist Tomogr 2003;27: 699–713.

37. Ducros A, Boukobza M, Porcher R, et al. The clinical and radiological spectrum of reversible cerebral vasoconstriction syndrome. A prospective series of 67 patients. Brain 2007;130:3091–101.

38. Keyserling HF, Provenzale JM. Atypical imaging findings in a near-fatal case of posterior reversible encephalopathy syndrome in a child. AJR Am J Roentgenol 2007;188:219–21.

39. Covarrubias DJ, Luetmer PH, Campeau NG. Posterior reversible encephalopathy syndrome: prognostic utility of quantitative diffusion-weighted MR images. AJNR Am J Neuroradiol 2002;23: 1038–48.

40. Brubaker LM, Smith JK, Lee YZ, et al. Hemodynamic and permeability changes in posterior reversible encephalopathy syndrome measured by dynamic susceptibility perfusion-weighted MR imaging. AJNR Am J Neuroradiol 2005;26:825–30.

41. Naidu K, Moodley J, Corr P, et al. Single photon emission and cerebral computerised tomographic scan and transcranial Doppler sonographic findings in eclampsia. Br J Obstet Gynaecol 1997;104:1165–72.

42. Schwartz R, Mulkern R, Vajapeyam S, et al. Catheter angiography, MR angiography, and MR perfusion in posterior reversible encephalopathy syndrome. AJNR Am J Neuroradiol 2009;30:E19 [author reply: E20].

43. Hecht JL, Ordi J, Carrilho C, et al. The pathology of eclampsia: An autopsy series. Hypertens Pregnancy 2017;36:259–68.

44. Sanders TG, Clayman DA, Sanchez-Ramos L, et al. Brain in eclampsia: MR imaging with clinical correlation. Radiology 1991;180:475–8.

45. Mintorovitch J, Moseley ME, Chileuitt L, et al. Comparison of diffusion- and T2-weighted MRI for the early detection of cerebral ischemia and reperfusion in rats. Magn Reson Med 1991;18:39–50.

46. Muttikkal TJ, Wintermark M. MRI patterns of global hypoxic-ischemic injury in adults. J Neuroradiol 2013;40:164–71.

47. Wijdicks EF, Campeau NG, Miller GM. MR imaging in comatose survivors of cardiac resuscitation. AJNR Am J Neuroradiol 2001;22:1561–5.

48. Ho ML, Rojas R, Eisenberg RL. Cerebral edema. AJR Am J Roentgenol 2012;199:W258–73.

49. Erdem A, Yasargil G, Roth P. Microsurgical anatomy of the hippocampal arteries. J Neurosurg 1993;79: 256–65.

50. Cianfoni A, Caulo M, Cerase A, et al. Seizure-induced brain lesions: a wide spectrum of variably reversible MRI abnormalities. Eur J Radiol 2013;82: 1964–72.

51. Casey SO, Truwit CL. Pontine reversible edema: a newly recognized imaging variant of hypertensive encephalopathy? AJNR Am J Neuroradiol 2000;21: 243–5.

52. Chang GY, Keane JR. Hypertensive brainstem encephalopathy: three cases presenting with severe brainstem edema. Neurology 1999;53:652–4.

53. de Seze J, Mastain B, Stojkovic T, et al. Unusual MR findings of the brain stem in arterial hypertension. AJNR Am J Neuroradiol 2000;21:391–4.

54. Bouri S, Thapar A, Shalhoub J, et al. Hypertension and the post-carotid endarterectomy cerebral hyperperfusion syndrome. Eur J Vasc Endovasc Surg 2011;41:229–37.

55. McKinney AM, Kieffer SA, Paylor RT, et al. Acute toxic leukoencephalopathy: potential for reversibility clinically and on MRI with diffusion-weighted and FLAIR imaging. AJR Am J Roentgenol 2009;193: 192–206.

56. Chen SP, Wang SJ. Hyperintense vessels: an early MRI marker of reversible cerebral vasoconstriction syndrome? Cephalalgia 2014;34:1038–9.

57. Ducros A, Fiedler U, Porcher R, et al. Hemorrhagic manifestations of reversible cerebral vasoconstriction syndrome: frequency, features, and risk factors. Stroke 2010;41:2505–11.

58. Singhal AB, Hajj-Ali RA, Topcuoglu MA, et al. Reversible cerebral vasoconstriction syndromes: analysis of 139 cases. Arch Neurol 2011;68: 1005–12.

59. Miller TR, Shivashankar R, Mossa-Basha M, et al. Reversible cerebral vasoconstriction syndrome, part 2: diagnostic work-up, imaging evaluation, and differential diagnosis. AJNR Am J Neuroradiol 2015;36:1580–8.

60. Linn J, Fesl G, Ottomeyer C, et al. Intra-arterial application of nimodipine in reversible cerebral vasoconstriction syndrome: a diagnostic tool in select cases? Cephalalgia 2011;31: 1074–81.

61. Singhal AB, Topcuoglu MA. Glucocorticoid-associated worsening in reversible cerebral vasoconstriction syndrome. Neurology 2017;88:228–36.

62. de Boysson H, Parienti JJ, Mawet J, et al. Primary angiitis of the CNS and reversible cerebral vasoconstriction syndrome: a comparative study. Neurology 2018;91:e1468–78.

63. Singhal AB, Topcuoglu MA, Fok JW, et al. Reversible cerebral vasoconstriction syndromes and primary angiitis of the central nervous system: clinical, imaging, and angiographic comparison. Ann Neurol 2016;79:882–94.

64. Kuker W, Gaertner S, Nagele T, et al. Vessel wall contrast enhancement: a diagnostic sign of cerebral vasculitis. Cerebrovasc Dis 2008;26:23–9.

65. Mandell DM, Matouk CC, Farb RI, et al. Vessel wall MRI to differentiate between reversible cerebral vasoconstriction syndrome and central nervous system vasculitis: preliminary results. Stroke 2012;43:860–2.

66. Rocha EA, Topcuoglu MA, Silva GS, et al. RCVS2 score and diagnostic approach for reversible cerebral vasoconstriction syndrome. Neurology 2019; 92:e639–47.

Adult Primary Brain Neoplasm, Including 2016 World Health Organization Classification

Kevin Yuqi Wang, MD[a], Melissa M. Chen, MD[b],
Christie M. Malayil Lincoln, MD[a],*

KEYWORDS

• WHO • Central nervous system • MR imaging • Adult primary neoplasm

KEY POINTS

- The 2016 update to the fourth edition of the World Health Organization central nervous system (CNS) tumor classification scheme represents a fundamental change in the manner in which tumors are classified and for the first time incorporates molecular parameters in addition to traditional microscopic features into the updated classification scheme.
- The most impactful changes involve classification of diffuse gliomas, with the incorporation of genetically defined features.
- Molecular markers of the genetically defined tumors are not only of diagnostic significance but also of prognostic value; examples include isocitrate dehydrogenase mutations and 1p/19q codeletions in astrocytomas and oligodendrogliomas, respectively.
- Imaging remains a mainstay modality in the diagnosis and management of adult primary CNS tumors, and familiarity with the new scheme is crucial for neuroradiologists to convey meaningful information to their referring colleagues.

INTRODUCTION

Updates in the 2016 World Health Organization Central Nervous System Tumor Classification

Primary central nervous system (CNS) tumors are the seventh most common adult neoplasm,[1] with an overall incidence rate of 23 cases per 100,000 people in the United States.[2] The most widely accepted classification scheme is based on the World Health Organization (WHO) classification of tumors of the CNS, currently in its fourth edition. For nearly the past century, the classification of CNS tumors was traditionally based on microscopic features, with the assumption that tumors could be classified according to histologic similarities based on the cells of origin (eg, astrocytomas originating from astrocytes or oligodendrogliomas originating from oligodendrocytes) and further subclassified based on their degree of cellular differentiation.[3] The past 2 decades of genetic and epigenetic research, however, have clarified the basis of tumorigenesis in a manner that has fundamentally altered the classification system. In the 2016 WHO classification, an update to the fourth edition represents a major paradigm shift in the manner in which CNS tumors are classified, for the first time integrating molecular parameters (genotypic) into the traditional microscopic features (phenotypic).[4]

The implications of this updated classification are both broad and deep. For example, prognoses

[a] Department of Radiology, Baylor College of Medicine, One Baylor Plaza, MS360, Houston, TX 77030, USA;
[b] Department of Diagnostic Radiology, Division of Diagnostic Imaging, The University of Texas MD Anderson Cancer Center, 1400 Pressler Street, Unit 1482, Houston, TX 77030, USA
* Corresponding author. One Baylor Plaza, MS360, Houston, TX 77030.
E-mail address: Christie.Lincoln@bcm.edu

Radiol Clin N Am 57 (2019) 1147–1162
https://doi.org/10.1016/j.rcl.2019.07.004

of certain tumors often correlate more strongly with molecular markers than with histologic grade (eg, isocitrate dehydrogenase [IDH] mutation status). The presence of molecular markers adds a level of objectivity and reproducibility conspicuously missing in a diagnostic process solely dependent on microscopic observation (eg, oligodendroglioma).[3] Reconciling discordance between genotypic and phenotypic parameters is now an issue. For example, a glioma that histologically and phenotypically appears astrocytic may possess a 1p/19q codeletion, a genotypic parameter that is almost always seen in oligodendrogliomas. Conversely, a tumor that histologically resembles oligodendroglioma may possess ATRX and TP53 mutations with an intact 1p and 19q, which are molecular signatures genotypically consistent with astrocytomas. Therefore, familiarity with the new classification scheme is critical for neuroradiologists to convey meaningful information for optimal collaborative disease management by radiation oncologists, neuropathologists, neuro-oncologists, and neurosurgeons.

Classification Considerations: Layered Diagnosis, Not Otherwise Specified, Not Elsewhere Classified

The concept of a layered diagnosis was introduced to assist in systematically diagnosing CNS tumors, incorporating both genotypic and phenotypic parameters into the diagnosis.[4,5] Layer 1 represents the integrated diagnosis, whereby a unifying summation of the molecular and microscopic data most accurately represents the diagnostic entity and can be generated only if information from all other layers are present. Layer 2 represents the histologic classification (eg, oligodendroglioma). Layer 3 presents the WHO grade (eg, WHO grade III). Layer 4 represents the molecular parameters (eg, 1p/19q codeletion). A layer 2 and 3 diagnosis can be made when no molecular data are available and is used to convey that a full, integrated layer 1 diagnosis is not possible.

The suffix not otherwise specified (NOS) is a designation in the 2016 WHO classification that denotes that the necessary molecular assays were unavailable or not performed at the facility to provide a layer 4 diagnosis for entities that may qualify for an integrated layer 1 diagnosis (eg, oligodendrogliomas, astrocytomas, or embryonal tumors). Therefore, the suffix conveys through the pathology report that the case has not been worked up to the necessary extent for a full, integrated layer 1 diagnosis. In contrast, the suffix, not elsewhere classified (NEC), is a designation used when molecular data analyses are performed and available, but the histologic (layer 2 and 3) and molecular (layer 4) data altogether are conflicting, therefore preventing a consensus diagnosis. It also may be used for increasingly well-described genetically defined entities for which there is no official recognition by the WHO classification scheme. This suffix is not yet codified in the 2016 WHO classification but likely will be utilized in the upcoming fifth edition.[6] For example, the NEC designation can be used in cases of histologically classic oligodendroglioma with an IDH-type molecular marker or histologically classic diffuse astrocytoma with molecular features of glioblastoma. NEC also can be used with new molecular entities, such as glioblastoma, *FGFR3-TACC3* fusion, which is resistant to conventional chemoradiation. It becomes important for the neuropathologist to identify these gliomas for inclusion in targeted therapeutic trials.[7]

Goals and Objectives

Although a comprehensive review of adult primary brain neoplasms based on the 2016 WHO classification is outside the scope of this article, the goal is to impart the readership with a working knowledge of the typical MR imaging findings of commonly encountered adult primary brain neoplasms and the relevant changes in 2016 WHO classification.

IMAGING TECHNIQUE AND CONSIDERATIONS

Imaging plays a major role as it represents the modern-day gross specimen. A differential diagnosis in order of probability can be formulated by scrutinizing all sources of information from a patient's clinical and demographic features (age, gender, and presenting symptoms/signs) to imaging findings: anatomic location, borders, and tissue characteristics of the lesion as well as the presence and pattern of contrast enhancement. A routine brain MR image offers conventional sequences used to evaluate brain tumors, including precontrast and postcontrast T1-weighted imaging (T1WI), T2-weighted imaging (T2WI), T2-weighted fluid-attenuated inversion recovery (FLAIR), diffusion-weighted imaging (DWI), and either gradient-recalled echo (GRE) or susceptibility-weighted imaging (SWI). Small field-of-view, thin-slice sagittal T2WI and sagittal postcontrast T1WI provide the best diagnostic value for tackling pineal region tumors. High-resolution T2WI, constructive interference in steady state, or fast imaging employing steady-state acquisition sequences of the cerebellopontine angle and internal auditory canal can be used to evaluate vestibular schwannomas. Small field-of-view, thin-slice precontrast and postcontrast images as well as postcontrast dynamic images are helpful when assessing sellar region neoplasms. Unless explicitly stated as otherwise, imaging findings discussed within this article are based on MR imaging.

PATHOLOGY AND IMAGING
Diffusely Infiltrating Gliomas

Gliomas represent a diverse and heterogeneous group of tumors. Based on the traditional phenotypic classification scheme, gliomas were thought to arise from a glial cell of origin. Therefore, subtypes of glial cells, such as astrocytes and oligodendrocytes, give rise to specific types of glioma, astrocytoma and oligodendroglioma, respectively.[1] Gliomas can be relatively circumscribed with a tendency toward benignity (eg, pleomorphic xanthoastrocytoma, pilocytic astrocytoma, and subependymal giant cell astrocytoma) or diffusely infiltrating with tendency toward malignancy (eg, diffuse astrocytoma and oligodendroglioma). Previously, in the 2007 WHO classification, all astrocytic tumors were grouped together. Due to differences in growth pattern and behavior between circumscribed and diffusely infiltrating gliomas, all diffusely infiltrating gliomas are now amassed into 1 category regardless of histologic subtype (eg, astrocytic or oligodendroglial).[4] Based on the 2016 WHO classification, diffusely infiltrating gliomas are composed of diffusely infiltrating astrocytomas, glioblastomas, and oligodendrogliomas.

Diffuse and anaplastic astrocytoma

After histologic confirmation and grading of diffusely infiltrating astrocytomas, including WHO grade II diffuse astrocytomas (not to be confused with the general term, diffusely infiltrating astrocytomas) and WHO grade III anaplastic astrocytomas (grade III), these tumors are further stratified by IDH mutations. Approximately 90% of grades II and III diffusely infiltrating astrocytomas are IDH-mutants.[1] Diffuse astrocytoma IDH–wild-type is such an uncommon diagnosis that reevaluation of an alternative diagnosis is often required.[4] Anaplastic astrocytoma IDH–wild-type also is uncommon, with most tumors sharing genetic features with those of glioblastoma IDH–wild-type.[4] Several recent studies have suggest minimal prognostic difference between grade II and grade III IDH-mutant astrocytomas[4] and further suggest that IDH status serves as a more accurate prognostic marker (IDH-mutant more favorable than IDH–wild-type) than WHO grading. At this time, however, the WHO grading scheme along with IDH status is retained; amendments are likely to occur in the next revision.[3]

On imaging, diffusely infiltrating astrocytomas are T2/FLAIR hyperintense masses that frequently arise from the cerebral hemispheres, with predilection for the frontal lobes. Despite their infiltrating growth pattern, they appear relatively circumscribed on imaging, tend to involve the underlying white matter, and are associated with characteristic cortical infiltration and gyral expansion. Both diffuse and anaplastic astrocytomas typically do not restrict on DWI and do not enhance with contrast. Enhancement is variably present in anaplastic astrocytomas (**Figs. 1** and **2**). Ultimately, no distinctive imaging features reliably distinguish astrocytomas by WHO grade and IDH status.

Glioblastoma

Glioblastoma is a grade IV diffusely infiltrating astrocytoma that is also further stratified by IDH

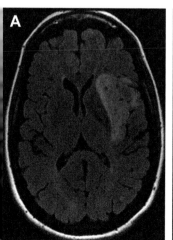
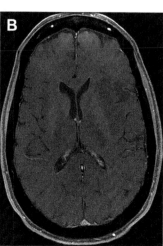

Fig. 1. Anaplastic astrocytoma, IDH-mutant on axial FLAIR and T1 postcontrast images manifests as a large cortical and subcortical nonenhancing area (*B*) of increasing signal (*A*) in the left lateral putamen, extreme capsule, insular cortex, and frontal operculum.

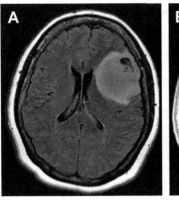
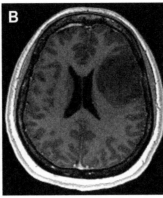

Fig. 2. A patient with diffuse astrocytoma, IDH-mutant with a larger nonenhancing area (B) of increased signal (A) in the left middle and inferior frontal gyri and operculum. Despite the size of the lesions in the index case, there is no subfalcine herniation or effacement of the lateral ventricles.

mutation status. Glioblastoma IDH–wild-type type arises de novo (clinically defined as primary glioblastoma), whereas glioblastoma IDH-mutant arises from a lower-grade IDH-mutant diffusely infiltrating astrocytoma (clinically defined as secondary glioblastoma).[8] Unlike astrocytoma, approximately 90% to 95% of glioblastomas are IDH–wild-type, tend to occur in patients greater than 55 years old, and portend a worse prognosis compared with IDH-mutants.[1,8] Despite arising de novo, glioblastoma IDH–wild-type shares other genetic alterations (eg, TERT promoter, EGFR amplification, and PTEN mutations) as well as clinical features with diffusely infiltrating astrocytoma IDH–wild-type,[1,4] perhaps reflecting a spectrum of the same entity.

The term, multifocal, glioblastoma, often is used when referring to multiple, seemingly separate foci of tumor that are connected by spread of disease via white matter tracts or cerebrospinal fluid. On the other hand, the term, multicentric glioblastoma, often is used when there is no obvious imaging finding demonstrating a connection among separate tumor foci. Glioblastoma IDH–wild-type

tumors classically demonstrate a thick, irregular rind of enhancing tumor, which histologically correlates with vascular proliferation. Centrally, a nonenhancing necrotic core typically preferentially involves the subcortical and deep white matter (Fig. 3) on postcontrast T1WI. T2/FLAIR sequences demonstrate a poorly marginated, heterogeneously hyperintense mass with mass effect and extensive vasogenic edema. Tumor invariably extends beyond the regions of enhancement, even beyond the extent of visible peritumoral edema, frequently along white matter tracts; this is referred to as microscopic invasion. The moniker, butterfly glioma, has been used when symmetric corpus callosum involvement is present. Nonenhancing tumor and vasogenic edema are virtually indistinguishable radiologically. Tumor heterogeneity is often due to a combination of necrosis and intratumoral hemorrhage; the latter is common and easily elucidated on GRE or SWI. Calcification and restricted diffusion are rare.

In contrast to astrocytomas, certain imaging findings may help distinguish glioblastoma

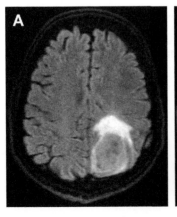
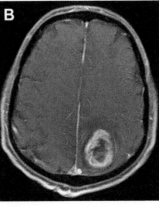

Fig. 3. Glioblastoma, IDH–wild-type exhibits a thick irregular ring of contrast enhancement (B) and central necrotic core with extensive vasogenic edema (A) in the left parietal lobe.

IDH-mutants from IDH–wild-type. Glioblastoma IDH-mutants preferentially involve the frontal lobes[4] and commonly have regions of nonenhancing tumor, not including the admixture of peritumoral edema/tumor.[1] The thick enhancing rind, intratumoral hemorrhage, and large centrally necrotic components, which are classic features of glioblastoma IDH–wild-type, are infrequent features in glioblastoma IDH-mutants (**Fig. 4**).

Oligodendroglioma
Oligodendroglioma (WHO grade II) and anaplastic oligodendroglioma (WHO grade III) share the same IDH gene family mutation as diffusely infiltrating astrocytomas. Oligodendrogliomas often are distinguished from astrocytomas by the presence of an additional 1p/19q codeletion. The less frequently encountered histologically classic oligodendroglioma with IDH–wild-type is given the diagnosis oligodendroglioma, NOS, after exclusion of other possible entities. In addition to its diagnostic value, the presence of a 1p/19q codeletion is prognostically significant in diffuse gliomas. Those with the codeletion receiving radiation followed by procarbazine, lomustine, and vincristine chemotherapy demonstrate significantly higher survival rates compared with those without the codeletion.[9–11] In contrast, similar to astrocytomas, the prognostic value of grading remains an issue, because several studies have failed to identify a difference in survival by WHO grade after IDH mutation status stratification.[12–14] Amendments to this histology-driven grading scheme may occur in the upcoming revision of the WHO classification scheme.[5]

Oligoastrocytomas were previously diagnosed based on the histologic admixture of both astrocytic and oligodendrolglial components; however, due to high interobserver variability, this criterion is strongly discouraged in the 2016 WHO classification. The vast majority of diffuse gliomas with histologic features of both astrocytic and oligodendroglial components can now be confidently classified as purely astrocytoma or oligodendroglioma based on genetic testing.[4]

On imaging, oligodendrogliomas occur predominantly supratentorially, with preference for the frontal lobes (50%–65%).[1] These tumors are relatively well defined, cortically based T2/FLAIR hyperintense masses with associated gyral expansion, occasional remodeling of the overlying calvarium, and frequent intratumoral coarse calcifications (**Fig. 5**). Preoperative calcification was found significantly predictive of the 1p/19q codeletion.[15] Peritumoral edema, hemorrhage, and necrosis are less common features. Similar to diffusely infiltrating astrocytomas, enhancement is inconsistent, with approximately 50% of cases manifesting some degree of enhancement, which is also unreliable in distinguishing grade II from grade III tumors.[1]

Diffuse midline glioma, H3 K27M-mutant
Diffuse midline gliomas, H3 K27M-mutant, are a new grade IV entity in the 2016 WHO classification. Although these tumors are classically seen in pediatric patients, recent studies demonstrate that they are not infrequently encountered in the adult population.[16,17] A recent case series of such tumors in adults reported the age range from ages 28 years to 81 years, with a median age of 52 years. Prognosis in the adult population is poor, similar to that in the pediatric population, with mean survival of 9.3 months.[16]

Typically found in the thalamus, pons, or hypothalamus, these tumors present as expansile T2/FLAIR hyperintense masses with variable enhancement (**Fig. 6**). Interestingly, 2 of the 4 criteria for pathologic diagnosis of this tumor are based on its imaging appearance. The tumors

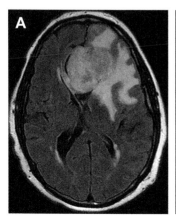
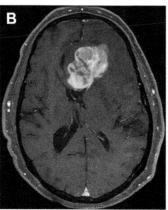

Fig. 4. Glioblastoma, IDH-mutant involves the left frontal lobe with more heterogeneous and solid areas of enhancement (*B*) and regions where there is nonenhancing tumor and vasogenic edema (*A*) in the white matter of the left frontal lobe and subinsular and extreme capsule region.

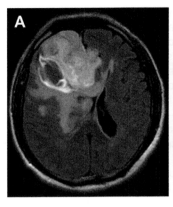
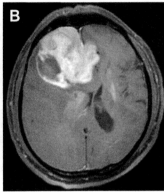

Fig. 5. Anaplastic oligodendroglioma, IDH-mutant, and 1p/19q-codeleted with well circumscribed, cortical-based, right frontal FLAIR hyperintense (*A*) and nearly homogenously enhancing tumor (*B*) with a small non-enhancing component and extensive vasogenic edema resulting in subfalcine herniation and partial effacement of the lateral ventricles. On CT (not shown), there was associated remodeling of the inner table of the right frontal calvarium and coarse calcifications within the tumor.

must appear diffuse and midline in addition to supporting the histologic diagnosis of glioma with the genetic mutation of H3 K27M.[18] Leptomeningeal dissemination has been reported.[16]

Ependymal Tumors

Ependymal tumors are a heterogeneous group of tumors that share histopathologic similarities despite arising from various anatomic sites across the neuroaxis.[1] The genetics and tumorigenesis of ependymomas are less well elucidated than in diffuse gliomas. Several studies have demonstrated limited value in the currently established histology-based classification and grading system.[19] Nevertheless, a few revisions were made in the 2016 WHO classification, because the presence of molecular markers to identify these subtypes is still forthcoming in most instances.[5,20,21] The exception is the ependymoma, *RELA* fusion-positive subtype, which comprises a majority of pediatric supratentorial tumors.[4,22] Moreover, with exception of myxopapillary ependymomas and subependymomas, a majority of ependymal tumors are seen in the pediatric population.

Subependymoma

Subependymomas are rare, slow-growing, WHO grade I tumors often found incidentally on imaging or autopsy in middle-aged to older adults.[1] If patients are symptomatic, it is usually secondary to obstructive hydrocephalus.

On imaging, approximately half of cases are found at the frontal horns of the lateral ventricles in close association with the septum pellucidum. The second most common location is in the fourth ventricle. They are well circumscribed, heterogeneously T2/FLAIR hyperintense masses that may expand the ventricle but otherwise demonstrate minimal mass effect (**Fig. 7**). When large, they may cause obstructive hydrocephalus. Other common imaging features include calcification and intratumoral cysts. These tumors show variable enhancement and rarely demonstrate restricted diffusion or hemorrhage.

Neuronal and Glioneuronal Tumors

Neuronal and mixed glioneuronal tumors are those that contain purely neurocytic or an admixture of neurocytic and glial elements, respectively.

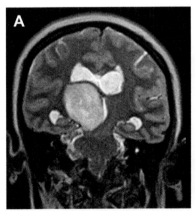
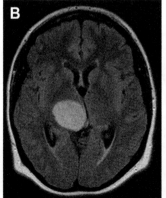
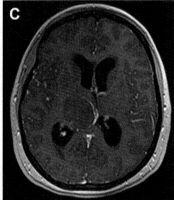

Fig. 6. A right thalamic diffuse midline glioma illustrates increased T2 (*A*) and FLAIR signal (*B*) and does not enhance (*C*). Despite the large size, there is no vasogenic edema; however, there is regional mass effect.

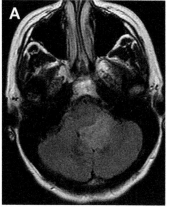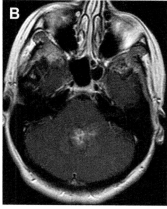

Fig. 7. A subependymoma expands the fourth ventricle and is a FLAIR hyperintense mass (*A*) with nonspecific, heterogeneous enhancement (*B*).

Glioneuronal tumors often are associated with clinical presentation of seizures, are lower in incidence than pure gliomas, and are associated with a better prognosis.[1] A majority of these neoplasms are designated WHO grade I.

Ganglioglioma and anaplastic ganglioglioma

Gangliogliomas are tumors histologically composed of a mix of neoplastic ganglion and glial elements. They are the most common glioneuronal tumor and the majority occur in children and young adults. As with many glioneuronal tumors, medically-refractory epilepsy is the typical presentation. The majority are benign, very indolent tumors and are, therefore, designated WHO grade I. Anaplastic gangliogliomas are relatively more rare, comprising only 8% to 10% of all gangliogliomas.[1] They are aggressive WHO grade III tumors; often, the glial component demonstrates malignant features histologically.[1]

On imaging, gangliogliomas arise most frequently in the temporal lobes as well defined, cortically based T2/FLAIR hyperintense lesions with solid and cystic components (**Fig. 8**). An enhancing mural nodule is typically seen arising from the cystic component of the tumor. Imaging features cannot reliably distinguish between benign and anaplastic gangliogliomas, although the latter may demonstrate more ill-defined margins and occur in more atypical locations.[1]

Gangliocytoma

Unlike gangliogliomas, gangliocytomas are benign neoplasms comprised exclusively of ganglion cells without glial elements, designated as WHO grade I. Similar to gangliogliomas, however, they occur frequently in children and young adults, often presenting with medically refractory epilepsy.

Imaging findings of gangliocytomas are indistinguishable from those of gangliogliomas. The typical location and imaging appearance is a cortically based T2/FLAIR hyperintense solid and cystic mass most frequently in the temporal lobe (**Fig. 9**). The solid components variably demonstrate intense homogeneous enhancement. Calcification within the solid components may be seen in approximately one-third of cases.[1]

Dysplastic cerebellar gangliocytoma

Also known as Lhermitte-Duclos disease, dysplastic cerebellar gangliocytoma is a slow-growing, infratentorial, benign, WHO grade I lesion of either neoplastic or hamartomatous nature. A majority of lesions are sporadic although may be seen in association with an autosomal-dominant phakomatosis, known as Cowden syndrome.[1]

As the name suggests, the lesion typically appears as a relatively well-defined, unilateral, expansile mass involving and replacing the cerebellar hemisphere and/or vermis. Mass effect and effacement of the fourth ventricle are common and can result in obstructive hydrocephalus. T2/FLAIR imaging demonstrates a characteristic gyriform and striated pattern of the lesion, reflecting the alternating intensities of the expanded and thickened cerebellar folia (**Fig. 10**). The tumor may restrict on DWI, perhaps reflecting its increased cellularity. Although enhancement is typically absent, enhancing vessels can be seen traversing the lesion and can be confirmed on T2WI, GRE, or SWI as signal void structures related to flow in the vasculature.

Rosette-forming glioneuronal tumor

Rosette-forming glioneuronal tumors are benign, slow-growing tumors of WHO grade I. The attribute, "of the fourth ventricle," has been removed from its name in the 2016 WHO classification, because it also occasionally may arise from the cerebellar vermis, cerebellar hemisphere, and

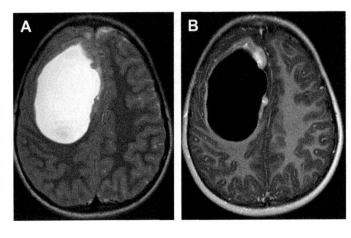

Fig. 8. A patient with right frontal cortical-based ganglioglioma that has a large FLAIR hyperintense cystic component (*A*), with solid peripheral enhancing mural nodules in the anterior and medial wall of the cyst (*B*).

pineal region, among other locations.[5] Rosette-forming glioneuronal tumors typically occur in young adults, with peak incidence in the third decade.[23]

Imaging typically demonstrates a markedly heterogeneous cystic and solid mass, mostly commonly located midline within the fourth ventricle or cerebellar vermis with variable presence of intratumoral hemorrhage, fluid-fluid levels, and calcification (**Fig. 11**). Heterogeneous and patchy enhancement is typical; CSF dissemination may occur.

Papillary glioneuronal tumor

Previously considered a ganglioglioma subtype, papillary glioneuronal tumors are now distinctly classified. They are slow-growing, WHO grade I tumors that predominantly affect young adults. Imaging findings are indistinguishable from gangliogliomas and include a well-defined mixed cystic

and solid mass, most frequently arising from the temporal lobes (**Fig. 12**).

Central neurocytoma

Central neurocytomas are benign, WHO grade II, intraventricular tumors with purely neurocytic elements, therefore originally thought to be a subtype of oligodendrogliomas. These tumors lack glial components, however, as well as the characteristic 1p/19q codeletion. Moreover, in the 2016 WHO classification, they are defined by the absence of IDH mutations,[5] further distinguishing them from oligodendrogliomas. They represent the most common primary intraventricular neoplasm of young to middle-aged adults.[1] Although slow-growing, central neurocytomas may result in sudden obstructive hydrocephalus due to their location.

On imaging, a well-defined heterogeneous, bubbly, T2/FLAIR hyperintense mass typically

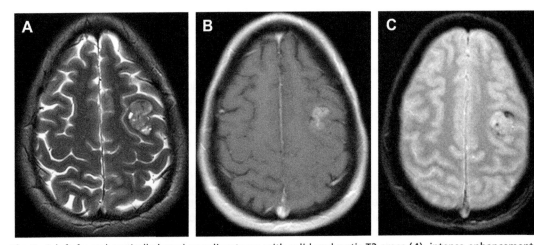

Fig. 9. A left frontal cortically based gangliocytoma with solid and cystic T2 areas (*A*), intense enhancement of the solid component (*B*), and areas of coarse calcification seen on gradient imaging (*C*).

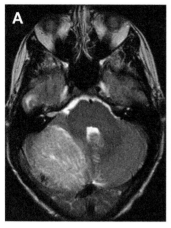
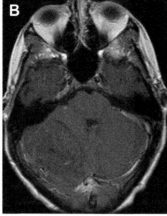

Fig. 10. An index case of right dysplastic cerebellar gangliocytoma that is nonenhancing (*B*), expansile, well defined, striated and gyriform pattern and replaces the entire right cerebellum (*A*). There is partial effacement of the fourth ventricle, and there are some enhancing vessels in the substance of this WHO grade I lesion (*B*).

arises from in the body of the lateral ventricle near the foramen of Monro, attached to the septum pellucidum[1] (**Fig. 13**). Calcification, intratumoral cysts, vascular flow-related signal void, and marked heterogeneous enhancement are common.

Pineal Gland Tumors

The approach to pineal gland tumors can be simplified into 2 broad categories: pineal parenchymal and germ cell tumors. Germ cell tumors are the most common group of pineal tumors, predominantly seen in the pediatric age group. Because they occupy a separate category in the WHO classification, they are described in the following section. Pineal parenchymal tumors arise from pinealocytes and comprise approximately 15% to 30% of all pineal gland tumors.[1] Though not the focus of this article, many other neoplastic and non-neoplastic entities may arise in the pineal region but originate outside of the pineal gland, evoking a diverse differential diagnosis.

Pineocytoma

Pineocytoma, one of the most common pineal parenchymal tumors, is a slow-growing, well-differentiated WHO grade I neoplasm. Small lesions often are asymptomatic, whereas large ones may cause obstructive hydrocephalus and Parinaud syndrome, defined as upward gaze palsy, pupillary light–near dissociation, and convergence retraction nystagmus.

On imaging, these tumors appear as T2/FLAIR hyperintense, well-defined, round or lobular masses with avid solid or rim enhancement and peripherally displaced calcifications (**Fig. 14**).[1] Intratumoral hemorrhage and cystic changes may be present. An entirely cystic pineocytoma may be indistinguishable from a non-neoplastic pineal cyst; differentiation may not be clinically significant because small lesions are observed with imaging.

Pineal parenchymal tumor of intermediate differentiation

Pineal parenchymal tumor of intermediate differentiation (PPTID), as the name suggests, is a tumor

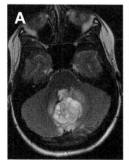
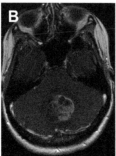
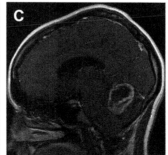
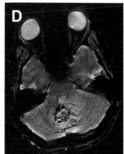

Fig. 11. A patient with Rosette-forming glioneuronal tumor manifests on brain MRI as a multiloculated T2 hyperintense cystic mass (*A*) with enhancing walls and septa on axial (*B*) and sagittal (*C*) postcontrast T1WI. It is centered in the posterior fourth ventricle and vermis, and there is also the presence of intratumoral hemorrhage, as shown on SWI (*D*).

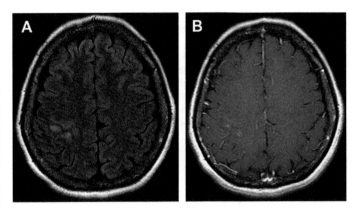

Fig. 12. A papillary glioneuronal tumor shows well circumscribed, cortical-based right parietal lobe FLAIR signal change (*A*) and wispy punctate and linear enhancement (*red arrow* [*B*]).

with intermediate prognosis between pineocytoma, and pineoblastoma PPTID may be designated a WHO grade II or III, although 1 study failed to find correlation with outcome.[24] Compared with pineocytomas, PPTIDs are larger in size, more heterogeneous, and overall more aggressive-appearing (see **Fig. 14**). Multiple cystic components may be present. Physiologic pineal calcifications may be engulfed or peripherally displaced by the mass. Obstructive hydrocephalus, splaying of the internal cerebral veins, and extension into the tectum, third and lateral ventricles, and thalamus are common.

Papillary tumor of the pineal region
Papillary tumors of the pineal region are rare WHO grade II or grade III neoplasms that do not arise

from the pineal gland but from the subcommissural organ of the third ventricle.[1] They are discussed due to their categorization with the primary parenchymal tumors in the 2016 WHO classification. The imaging findings are indistinguishable from those of PPTID.

Meningiomas

Meningiomas are the most common primary intracranial neoplasms. This tumor category includes typical meningiomas, which are benign WHO grade I tumors, and meningioma variants, which include tumors with more aggressive clinical behavior, such as WHO grade II atypical meningiomas and WHO grade III anaplastic meningiomas.[1] Although previously considered a staging feature, brain invasion in the 2016 WHO

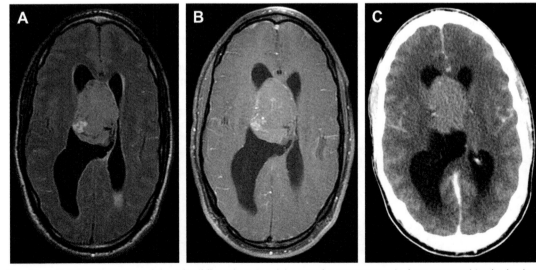

Fig. 13. A FLAIR hyperintense (*A*) and mildly enhancing (*B*) central neurocytoma is demonstrated in the body of the right lateral ventricle with bowing the septum pellucidum to the left and obstructive hydrocephalus. The axial head CT with contrast shows mild enhancement of the large right lateral ventricle lesion and obstructive hydrocephalus (*C*).

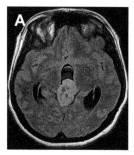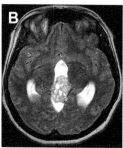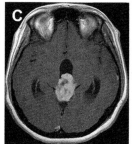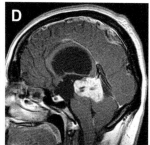

Fig. 14. A PPTID displays heterogeneous signal intensity lesion on axial FLAIR (*A*) and T2WI (*B*), heterogeneous enhancement on axial (*C*) and sagittal (*D*) postcontrast T1WI, and resultant regional mass effect on the tectal plate with effacement of the cerebral aqueduct and obstructive hydrocephalus.

classification is now considered a grading feature and a histologic criterion, which in itself may establish the diagnosis of WHO grade II atypical meningioma.[4,5]

Typical meningioma

Typical meningiomas account for approximately 95% of all meningiomas.[1] They are benign, WHO grade I tumors most commonly located along the convexity, parasagittal region, or the sphenoid ridge, although they may occur almost anywhere within the CNS (eg, orbits, sinuses, calvarium, ventricles, or pineal region). They are seen most commonly in middle-aged to older adults, with female predominance. Ionizing radiation is a risk factor. A majority of tumors are asymptomatic, incidental, and indolent. Despite their WHO grade I classification, metastases have been rarely reported.[25]

Typical imaging findings include an extra-axial, dural-based, well-defined, markedly homogeneously enhancing mass (Fig. 15A, B). Tumor shape may be round, lobulated, or flat (en plaque). On CT, a vast majority are hyperdense and hyperostosis of the overlying calvarium may be present.

Peritumoral edema of the underlying brain parenchyma is present in approximately half of cases irrespective of size or grade.[1] Calcification is seen in one-quarter of cases (see Fig. 15C). Intratumoral cysts and hemorrhage are rare. Signal void structures may be present, reflecting tumor vascularity. If present, a dural tail, representing reactive dura, is suggestive of, but not specific for, meningioma.

Atypical meningioma

Atypical meningiomas are WHO grade II tumors diagnosed histologically by the presence of greater than or equal to 4 mitotic figures per high-power field, brain invasion, or on the basis of additive criteria of 3 out of 5 histologic findings.[4] They are associated with higher recurrence rates compared with typical meningiomas.[1]

Unlike typical meningiomas, atypical meningiomas more frequently exhibit ill-defined margins, invasion, and destruction of overlying calvarium or invasion of the underlying parenchyma (Fig. 16). The absence of such findings does not exclude atypical meningioma; brain invasion inconspicuous on imaging may be present on

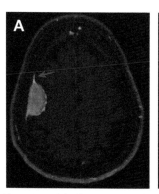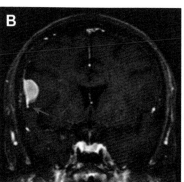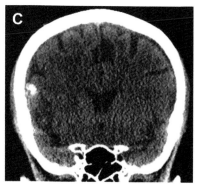

Fig. 15. A right frontoparietal convexity typical meningioma on brain MR imaging shows homogenous enhancement with dural tail (*red arrow*) on axial (*A*) and coronal (*B*) postcontrast T1WI. There are coarse calcifications associated with the tumor as seen on the noncontrast coronal head CT (*C*).

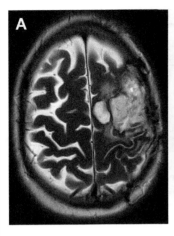
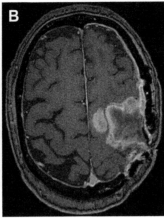

Fig. 16. Atypical meningioma shows irregular margins and invasion of the left frontal and precentral gyrus with associated vasogenic edema (*A*) and irregular enhancement after contrast administration (*B*). There is evidence of prior left frontoparietal craniotomy from prior resection.

histology. Unfortunately, no imaging feature reliably distinguishes typical meningioma from its more aggressive variants, albeit typical meningiomas are statistically far more common. The mushrooming sign, representing tumor extending away from the more central predominant component of the mass, has been associated with higher grade meningiomas.[26]

Anaplastic meningioma

Also known as malignant meningiomas, anaplastic meningiomas are WHO grade III tumors whose diagnosis is based on overt histologic features of malignancy (eg, pleomorphism and high mitotic rates). The prognosis is poor, with low recurrence-free and overall survival rates. Imaging findings overlap with those of atypical meningiomas, including the mushrooming appearance.

Nerve Sheath Tumors

A vast majority of intracranial and skull base nerve sheath tumors are benign, rare (with the exception of vestibular schwannomas), and associated with cranial nerves (CNs). Hybrid nerve sheath tumors (a histologic combination of schwannomas, neurofibromas, and perineuriomas) and melanotic schwannomas have been included as new entities in the 2016 WHO classification.[4] Hybrid nerve sheath tumors are seen more commonly in the body than in the CNS. Two subtypes of malignant peripheral nerve sheath tumors (MPNSTs) now exist: epithelioid MPNSTs and MPNSTs with perineurial differentiation.[4]

Schwannoma

Schwannomas are benign, WHO grade I, slow-growing tumors composed of well-differentiated Schwann cells; they may arise from CN III through CN XII or any peripheral nerve. Approximately 95% of schwannomas arise from CN VIII; CN V is the second most common CN of origin,[1] with involvement of the remaining CNs comprising a small minority of cases. Multinodular or plexiform schwannomas are tumors with multiple consecutive lesions arising along a nerve fascicle along the neck, trunk, and extremities.

Imaging reveals a well-defined extra-axial, T2/FLAIR hyperintense, and avidly homogeneously

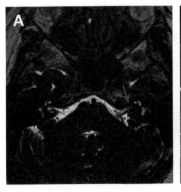
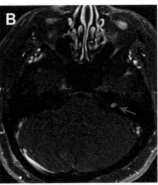

Fig. 17. A small schwannoma is seen as a filling defect on heavily T2 imaging through the internal auditory canals (*red arrow* [*A*]) and homogenously enhances (*red arrow* [*B*]).

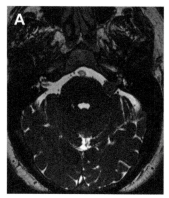
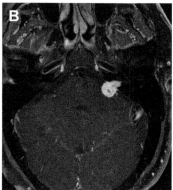

Fig. 18. A large schwannoma shows slight T2 hyperintensity on heavily T2-weighted sequence through the internal auditory canal (*A*) and near-complete homogenous enhancement (*B*). There is a focus of hypoenhancement in the lesion representing cystic degenerative change.

or heterogeneously enhancing mass near or arising from a CN. In contrast to meningiomas, intratumoral calcification and dural tails are rare, whereas microhemorrhage is characteristic for schwannomas. Approximately 15% of tumors have intratumoral cysts.[1] Small intracanalicular vestibular schwannomas present simply as round or fusiform filling defects within the normal bright CSF on heavily T2WI (**Fig. 17**). Larger vestibular schwannomas may project out of the porus acusticus into the cerebellopontine angle with potential mass effect on the adjacent pons, middle cerebellar peduncle, and fourth ventricle (**Fig. 18**).

Melanotic schwannoma

Approximately 10% of melanotic schwannomas demonstrate malignant behavior. Moreover, approximately 50% of the psammomatous subtype melanotic schwannomas are genetically distinct from conventional schwannomas, in which they are associated with Carney complex and PRKAR1A gene mutation.[27] In light of these findings, melanotic schwannomas are now classified as a distinct entity rather than as a variant.

These tumors most commonly occur in paraspinal and extraneural locations.[1] The presence of melanin accounts for the hyperintense T1 and hypointense T2 signal of these lesions; enhancement is variable.

Neurofibroma

Neurofibromas are WHO grade I neoplasms that can occur anywhere in the dermis or subcutis of the body and rarely along CNs. Multiple neurofibromas and/or plexiform neurofibromas occur in neurofibromatosis type 1 (NF-1). Solitary and sporadic neurofibromas may occur outside of the NF-1 setting and affect patients of all ages.

On imaging, sporadic neurofibromas of the head and neck most frequently present as focal, homogeneously enhancing, well-defined round or ovoid scalp masses that abut and remodel the underlying calvarium (**Fig. 19**A). In contrast, plexiform neurofibromas present as extensive, infiltrating, heterogeneously enhancing soft tissue masses invading and deforming the scalp, parotid gland, or orbit with surround bony remodeling and expansion (see **Fig. 19**B).

Malignant peripheral nerve sheath tumors

MPNSTs are rare malignancies most frequently involving spinal and peripheral nerves, and rarely CNs, arising either de novo or via malignant degeneration of a neurofibroma. Those arising from a peripheral nerve are strongly associated with NF-1.

Small MPNSTs may be radiologically indistinguishable from schwannomas or sporadic fibromas. Large MPNSTs have similar infiltrating

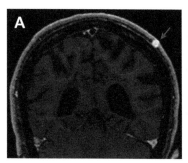
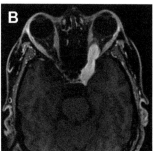

Fig. 19. A patient with a left parietal small scalp neurofibroma is seen on the coronal postcontrast image (*red arrow* [*A*]). A postcontrast axial T1 in a different patient shows a homogenously enhancing neurofibroma of left CN III (*B*).

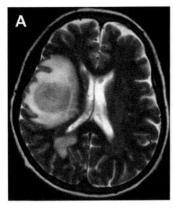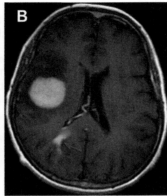

Fig. 20. Diffuse large B-cell lymphoma in this immunocompetent patient exhibits heterogeneous right corona radiata lesion with extensive vasogenic edema (*A*) and homogenous enhancement (*B*). There is a smaller heterogeneous T2 lesion (*A*) in the right splenium of the corpus callosum that homogenously enhances (*red arrow* [*B*]) and represents a satellite tumor.

appearances as plexiform neurofibromas but are more likely to demonstrate frank bone invasion and destruction. Sudden rapid enlargement and painfulness of a previous plexiform neurofibroma raises suspicion malignant degeneration. The optimal way to distinguish between MPNSTs from the benign counterpart is with 2-deoxy-2-(18F)fluoro-D-glucose PET where a standardized uptake value of greater than 3 indicates MPNST.[28]

Lymphoma and Mesenchymal Tumors

Expansion of entities in the classification of systemic lymphomas over the past decade has been followed by similar updates in 2016 CNS WHO classification.[4] Greater than 95% of CNS lymphomas, however, remain diffuse large B-cell lymphomas, which are the specific type discussed in this article.[1] A brief discussion of a particular mesenchymal tumor, solitary fibrous tumors (SFTs), is also provided, given changes in the 2016 WHO classification.

Diffuse large B-cell lymphoma
On imaging, up to three-fourths of diffuse large B-cell lymphomas contact the CSF via the ependymal or pial surface.[1] Periventricular white matter and deep gray nuclei are the most common locations; involvement of the subependyma and corpus callosum is not infrequent. Lesions characteristically homogenously enhance, restrict on DWI, and are hyperdense on CT (**Fig. 20**), correlating to the densely packed cells angiocentric pattern of tumor cells within and around blood vessels. By comparison, multifocality, necrosis, ring or heterogeneous enhancement, and intratumoral hemorrhage may be seen in immunocompromised patients, including those with human immunodeficiency virus, making such tumors indistinguishable from glioblastoma on imaging.

Solitary fibrous tumor/hemangiopericytoma
It is now apparent that SFTs and hemangiopericytomas are very similar, if not the same entity.[29,30] Neuropathologists now join the rest of soft tissue pathologists in using the term, *SFT*, but retain the term, *hemangiopericytoma*, to create the combined moniker, *SFT/hemangiopericytoma*, for continuity. SFTs represent a continuum of mesenchymal tumors with varying cellularity notorious for their aggressive behavior, recurrence, and metastases, which may be designated WHO grade I, II, or III.

Low-grade SFTs are well-defined, extra-axial, dural-based, heterogeneously intense, avidly enhancing masses that mimic typical meningiomas and most commonly occur at the posterior falx or tentorium. High-grade SFTs mimic aggressive meningiomas; however, dural tails, hyperostosis, and intratumoral calcification typically are absent.

SUMMARY

The unprecedented use of molecular parameters and creation of genetically defined parameters to establish brain tumor diagnoses in the 2016 WHO classification is a major paradigm shift. Major paradigm restructuring resulted in classifying diffuse gliomas, such as astrocytomas, oligodendrogliomas, and glioblastomas, as genetically defined entities. Molecular markers not only are of diagnostic significance but also are of prognostic value. These more objectively defined entities allow for more accurate diagnoses, therapies, stratification, and recruitment within clinical trials, and categorization in epidemiologic studies. Imaging remains a mainstay modality in the diagnosis and management of these entities, and familiarity with the new classification scheme, therefore, is crucial for neuroradiologists to communicate meaningfully with radiation oncologists, neuropathologists, neuro-oncologists, and neurosurgeons.

REFERENCES

1. Osborn AG, Hedlund GL, Salzman KL. Osborn's brain. 2nd edition. Salt Lake City (UT): Elsevier; 2018.

2. Ostrom QT, Gittleman H, Truitt G, et al. CBTRUS statistical report: primary brain and other central nervous system tumors diagnosed in the United States in 2011-2015. Neuro Oncol 2018;20(suppl_4):iv1–86.

3. Komori T. The 2016 WHO classification of tumours of the central nervous system: the major points of revision. Neurol Med Chir (Tokyo) 2017;57(7): 301–11.

4. Louis DN, Perry A, Reifenberger G, et al. The 2016 World Health Organization classification of tumors of the central nervous system: a summary. Acta Neuropathol 2016;131(6):803–20.

5. Banan R, Hartmann C. The new WHO 2016 classification of brain tumors-what neurosurgeons need to know. Acta Neurochir (Wien) 2017;159(3): 403–18.

6. Louis DN, Wesseling P, Paulus W, et al. cIMPACT-NOW update 1: not otherwise specified (NOS) and not elsewhere classified (NEC). Acta Neuropathol 2018;135(3):481–4.

7. Bielle F, Di Stefano AL, Meyronet D, et al. Diffuse gliomas with FGFR3-TACC3 fusion have characteristic histopathological and molecular features. Brain Pathol 2018;28(5):674–83.

8. Johnson DR, Guerin JB, Giannini C, et al. 2016 updates to the WHO brain tumor classification system: what the radiologist needs to know. Radiographics 2017;37(7):2164–80.

9. van den Bent MJ, Brandes AA, Taphoorn MJ, et al. Adjuvant procarbazine, lomustine, and vincristine chemotherapy in newly diagnosed anaplastic oligodendroglioma: long-term follow-up of EORTC brain tumor group study 26951. J Clin Oncol 2013;31(3): 344–50.

10. Cairncross JG, Wang M, Jenkins RB, et al. Benefit from procarbazine, lomustine, and vincristine in oligodendroglial tumors is associated with mutation of IDH. J Clin Oncol 2014;32(8):783–90.

11. Buckner JC, Shaw EG, Pugh SL, et al. Radiation plus procarbazine, CCNU, and vincristine in low-grade glioma. N Engl J Med 2016;374(14): 1344–55.

12. Weller M, Weber RG, Willscher E, et al. Molecular classification of diffuse cerebral WHO grade II/III gliomas using genome- and transcriptome-wide profiling improves stratification of prognostically distinct patient groups. Acta Neuropathol 2015; 129(5):679–93.

13. Suzuki H, Aoki K, Chiba K, et al. Mutational landscape and clonal architecture in grade II and III gliomas. Nat Genet 2015;47(5):458–68.

14. Olar A, Wani KM, Alfaro-Munoz KD, et al. IDH mutation status and role of WHO grade and mitotic index in overall survival in grade II-III diffuse gliomas. Acta Neuropathol 2015;129(4):585–96.

15. Saito T, Muragaki Y, Maruyama T, et al. Calcification on CT is a simple and valuable preoperative indicator of 1p/19q loss of heterozygosity in supratentorial brain tumors that are suspected grade II and III gliomas. Brain Tumor Pathol 2016;33(3): 175–82.

16. Kleinschmidt-DeMasters BK, Mulcahy Levy JM. H3 K27M-mutant gliomas in adults vs. children share similar histological features and adverse prognosis. Clin Neuropathol 2018;37 (2018)(2): 53–63.

17. Ebrahimi A, Skardelly M, Schuhmann MU, et al. High frequency of H3 K27M mutations in adult midline gliomas. J Cancer Res Clin Oncol 2019; 145(4):839–50.

18. Louis DN, Giannini C, Capper D, et al. cIMPACT-NOW update 2: diagnostic clarifications for diffuse midline glioma, H3 K27M-mutant and diffuse astrocytoma/anaplastic astrocytoma, IDH-mutant. Acta Neuropathol 2018;135(4):639–42.

19. Tihan T, Zhou T, Holmes E, et al. The prognostic value of histological grading of posterior fossa ependymomas in children: a Children's Oncology Group study and a review of prognostic factors. Mod Pathol 2008;21(2):165–77.

20. Pajtler KW, Witt H, Sill M, et al. Molecular classification of ependymal tumors across all CNS compartments, histopathological grades, and age groups. Cancer Cell 2015;27(5):728–43.

21. Mack SC, Witt H, Piro RM, et al. Epigenomic alterations define lethal CIMP-positive ependymomas of infancy. Nature 2014;506(7489):445–50.

22. Parker M, Mohankumar KM, Punchihewa C, et al. C11orf95-RELA fusions drive oncogenic NF-kappaB signalling in ependymoma. Nature 2014; 506(7489):451–5.

23. Yang C, Fang J, Li G, et al. Histopathological, molecular, clinical and radiological characterization of rosette-forming glioneuronal tumor in the central nervous system. Oncotarget 2017;8(65): 109175–90.

24. Yu T, Sun X, Wang J, et al. Twenty-seven cases of pineal parenchymal tumours of intermediate differentiation: mitotic count, Ki-67 labelling index and extent of resection predict prognosis. J Neurol Neurosurg Psychiatry 2016;87(4):386–95.

25. Simonetti G, Terreni MR, DiMeco F, et al. Letter to the editor: lung metastasis in WHO grade I meningioma. Neurol Sci 2018;39(10):1781–3.

26. Shapir J, Coblentz C, Malanson D, et al. New CT finding in aggressive meningioma. AJNR Am J Neuroradiol 1985;6(1):101–2.

27. Carney JA. Psammomatous melanotic schwannoma. A distinctive, heritable tumor with special associations, including cardiac myxoma and the Cushing syndrome. Am J Surg Pathol 1990;14(3): 206–22.

28. Vezina G. Neuroimaging of phakomatoses: overview and advances. Pediatr Radiol 2015;45(Suppl 3): S433–42.

29. Robinson DR, Wu YM, Kalyana-Sundaram S, et al. Identification of recurrent NAB2-STAT6 gene fusions in solitary fibrous tumor by integrative sequencing. Nat Genet 2013;45(2):180–5.

30. Chmielecki J, Crago AM, Rosenberg M, et al. Whole-exome sequencing identifies a recurrent NAB2-STAT6 fusion in solitary fibrous tumors. Nat Genet 2013;45(2):131–2.

Primary Neoplasms of the Pediatric Brain

Camilo Jaimes, MD*, Tina Young Poussaint, MD

KEYWORDS

• Pediatric brain tumors • MR imaging • Diffusion • Perfusion • Spectroscopy • Neuroimaging

KEY POINTS

- Pediatric brain tumors differ from adult brain tumors in their epidemiology, genetics, molecular characteristics, and imaging appearance.
- Low-grade gliomas are the most common central nervous system tumor in childhood. They are characterized by mutations in the mitogen-activated protein kinase pathway. The most common mutation is the KIAA1549:BRAF fusion, present in a large majority of pilocytic astrocytomas, followed by the BRAFV600E point deletion, which occurs in several histologic types of low-grade gliomas.
- Histone variants are common in pediatric supratentorial and infratentorial high-grade gliomas. Hemispheric tumors harbor H3.3G34R/V mutations, whereas midline tumors have H3.3K27M and H3.1K27M mutations.
- Medulloblastomas are divided into unique molecular subgroups with differing prognosis and imaging features.
- Ependymomas are divided into 2 molecular groups, Ependymoma A and B. Ependymoma A accounts for the large majority of tumors and demonstrates a CPG island methylated phenotype.

INTRODUCTION

Primary brain tumors are an important cause of morbidity and mortality in children and adolescents. These tumors represent the most common solid tumor of childhood, second only to leukemia in incidence. According to the 2018 report from the Central Brain Tumor Registry of the United States, the incidence of brain tumors is approximately 5.65 per 100,000 in children 0 to 14 years and 6.19 per 100,000 in adolescents 15 to 19 years.[1,2] In view of their high incidence, brain tumors constitute the most common cause of cancer-related death in children 0 to 14 years of age and the second most common cause in adolescents 15 to 19 years old.[2,3]

Understanding differences in the histology, molecular genetics, and prognosis between tumors that affect children and those that occur in adults is critical. These differences fundamentally impact diagnostic considerations. For example, the incidence of high-grade glial tumors is much lower in children relative to adults.[2,3] However, leptomeningeal dissemination occurs more frequently in children, often requiring screening of the entire neuroaxis at presentation.[4] Assessment of treatment response is also difficult in pediatric patients, owing to the heterogeneous and unique molecular landscape of pediatric brain tumors, emerging new therapies such as checkpoint inhibitors, and the background of development-related changes.[5] To address this, a multidisciplinary working group recently proposed a set of guidelines to standardize

Disclosures: None.
Department of Radiology, Boston Children's Hospital, Harvard Medical School, 300 Longwood Avenue, Boston, MA 02115, USA
* Corresponding author.
E-mail address: Camilo.jaimescobos@childrens.harvard.edu

Radiol Clin N Am 57 (2019) 1163–1175
https://doi.org/10.1016/j.rcl.2019.06.004

response assessment in pediatric neurooncology (RAPNO). The first set of these guidelines, aimed at evaluating medulloblastoma (MB) and other cerebrospinal fluid (CSF) disseminating tumors, includes criteria on craniospinal MR imaging, clinical examination, and CSF cytology.[6,7] Additional RAPNO working groups are currently in place for low-grade gliomas (LGG), high-grade gliomas (HGG), and diffuse intrinsic pontine glioma. A review of detailed recommendations of these groups is beyond the scope of this article.

This article discusses the imaging approach to pediatric brain tumors, highlighting technical considerations unique to imaging children, and emerging techniques that address pediatric-specific challenges. The second part of the article discusses a subgroup of common primary pediatric brain tumors, emphasizing novel molecular insights into tumor subgroups and their clinical implications.

IMAGING MODALITIES
Computed Tomography

In the acute setting, computed tomography (CT) is often used as the initial imaging modality. Findings that can be diagnostically evaluated with CT include acute intracranial hemorrhage, mineralization, hydrocephalus, mass effect, midline shift, and the presence of vasogenic edema.[8] Once the diagnosis of an intracranial mass is made or suspected, MR imaging is typically required for definitive lesion characterization. Because of the unique sensitivity of children to ionizing radiation, low-dose protocols that adhere to the ALARA ("as low as reasonably achievable") principle should be followed.[9,10]

MR Imaging

MR imaging is the modality of choice to diagnose a brain tumor, delineate its anatomic extent, and narrow the differential diagnosis. Although protocols vary among institutions, they typically include a series of multiplanar sequences that examine T1 and T2 signal characteristics, vascularity, and tissue diffusivity.[6] **Table 1** summarizes the routine brain tumor protocol at Boston Children's Hospital. They use 3-dimensional (3D) T1-sampling perfection with application of optimized contrasts using different flip angle evolution (SPACE) as the main contrast-enhanced sequence because the "black-blood" effect of this spin-echo–based sequence facilitates detection of pathologic leptomeningeal enhancement.[11] Postcontrast fluid-attenuated inversion recovery (FLAIR) imaging has been proposed as an adjunct to T1-SPACE imaging for detection of subtle leptomeningeal abnormalities and should be considered in cases of equivocal findings on T1-SPACE sequences.[7,11]

Table 1	
Sequences of routine brain tumor protocol at Boston Children's Hospital	
Sequence	**Role/Findings**
Sagittal T1 MPRAGE	• Anatomic detail (gray-white matter contrast) • Blood products
Axial T2	• Cytotoxic and vasogenic edema • Tumor nodules and masses • Infiltrative tumor • Ventricular contour and sulcal effacement
Axial (T2) FLAIR with fat suppression	• Cytotoxic edema • Gliosis • Infiltrative tumor • Transependymal edema
Axial diffusion tensor imaging	• Tissue cellularity • Demonstration of white matter tracts • ADC histogram metrics for treatment response and prognosis • Devitalized tissue and infection (postoperative)
Sagittal postcontrast T1-SPACE	• Enhancing intraaxial components • Leptomeningeal dissemination of tumor
Optional: DCE perfusion	• Evaluation of blood-brain permeability and tumor microvasculature

Additional sequences are occasionally acquired as problem-solving tools or to clarify specific findings. For example, susceptibility-weighted images (SWI) help identify hemorrhagic and mineralized components; after surgery and treatment, SWI helps characterize blood products and outline treatment-related changes, such as postradiation vasculopathy.[6,12] Occasionally, 3D cisternographic sequences (eg, heavily T2-weighted sequences such as T2-SPACE or constructive interference steady state) can be used to delineate the interface between CSF and parenchyma, which facilitates the assessment of the contour of cranial nerves and CSF recesses for leptomeningeal tumor spread.[13]

Given the high prevalence of CSF-seeding tumors, postcontrast imaging of the entire neuroaxis is advised on initial presentation.[6] At the authors' institution, they perform sagittal 2-dimensional T1-weighted sequences through the entire spine and acquire axial images if suspicious findings are identified. In cases of nonenhancing primary tumors, addition of 3D cisternographic sequences through the spine or RESOLVE-DWI can be used to increase sensitivity.[14,15]

Advanced imaging

MR imaging assessment of perfusion can be performed with or without intravenous contrast. Dynamic susceptibility contrast perfusion relies on T2* properties of gadolinium and estimates cerebral blood flow (CBF), cerebral blood volume (CBV), and mean transit time based on signal loss related to the paramagnetic effect of gadolinium contrast.[16] Dynamic contrast-enhanced (DCE) perfusion is an alternative approach that relies on quantification of T1-shortening associated with gadolinium chelates. DCE uses pharmacokinetic models to characterize microvascular permeability.[17] Arterial spin labeling is a noncontrast MR imaging perfusion technique that uses a magnetic pulse to tag incoming blood into the brain and subsequently measures signal from the labeled spins to estimate CBF as they traverse the brain capillaries.[18]

Magnetic resonance spectroscopy (MRS) can aid in the evaluation of pediatric brain tumors by providing metabolic information complementary to neuroanatomical imaging.[19] MRS is typically performed as 2 independent acquisitions using a short time-to-echo (TE) (30 milliseconds) and an intermediate TE (135 milliseconds).[20] The intermediate TE acquisition demonstrates the peaks from molecules with long T2 decay times, which constitute the dominant peaks in the MR spectrum, including *N*-acetyl aspartate (NAA), choline (Cho), and creatine (Cr). In addition to these large peaks, the short TE acquisition also demonstrates peaks from smaller molecules with shorter T2-decay times, such as taurine, glutamine and glutamate, myoinositol, and alanine.[20]

BRAIN TUMORS
Supratentorial Tumors

Tumors of the cerebral hemispheres, corpus callosum, and other intraaxial supratentorial structures account for approximately 20% of brain tumors in children 0 to 14 years of age, with the highest incidence in infants, where they account for 30% of lesions. Supratentorial brain tumors are extremely diverse and include LGG, HGG, and embryonal tumors, among others.[3]

Low-grade gliomas

Pediatric LGG, classified as World Health Organization (WHO) I and II, are the most common central nervous tumor in children.[21] LGGs can be broadly divided into 3 large categories: astrocytic tumors (eg, pilocytic and pilomyxoid astrocytomas),

oligodendrocytic tumors, and neuronal/glioneuronal tumors (eg, ganglioglioma, dysembryoblastic neuroepithelial tumor). The single most common histologic subtype of LGG in pediatric patients is the pilocytic astrocytoma.[22] Although the cerebellum is the most common site of occurrence, nearly half of the cases involve supratentorial structures, including the cerebral hemispheres, deep cerebral structures, and the optic pathway.[22] By virtue of their predisposition to develop tumors, subjects with neurofibromatosis type 1 (NF-1) have a higher incidence of LGGs.

Imaging appearance varies largely across histologic and molecular subgroups of LGGs. In general, the tumors are well circumscribed, have little or no surrounding vasogenic edema, and demonstrate increased diffusivity. Many, but not all LGGs enhance avidly, and it is important to emphasize that the presence of enhancement does not portend a worse prognosis or higher tumor grade. Pilocytic astrocytomas serve as a good example. In the supratentorial compartment, these tumors can either present as a cyst with an avidly enhancing nodule or a solid enhancing nodule.[23] MRS features can be reminiscent of those seen in high-grade neoplasms, with an elevation of Cho, a decrease in NAA, and lactate peaks.[24] CBV in the solid components of the tumor is usually lower than that of high-grade neoplasms, although rarely the values may overlap.[24] A unique presentation of a suprasellar pilocytic astrocytoma occurs when the tumor involves the hypothalamus and optic pathway, known as an optic pathway glioma (OPG) (**Fig. 1**). Although most of these cases are sporadic, up to a third are seen in patients with NF-1. NF-1 OPGs show a higher frequency of prechiasmatic involvement, present at a younger age, and have a better prognosis than those in patients without NF-1.[25]

Other LGGs with avid enhancement include pilocytic xanthoastrocytoma (PXA) and ganglioglioma/ganglioneuroma. PXAs account for approximately 1% of all astrocytic LGGs and typically demonstrate an avidly enhancing mural nodule with an associated cyst. These tumors are usually cortical or juxtacortical with occasional scalloping of the adjacent inner calvarial table, and frequent involvement of the temporal lobes (39%), frontal lobes (18%), and parietal lobes (14%).[26] Gangliogliomas also present with an enhancing nodule associated with a cyst; these tumors overwhelmingly affect the temporal lobes (up to 80% of cases), explaining their high association with refractory epilepsy (**Fig. 2**). The appearance of ganglioglioma is similar to that of PXA, although gangliogliomas are more often associated with calcifications.[27]

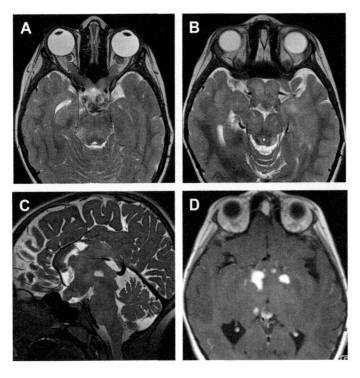

Fig. 1. A 5-year-old boy with NF-1 and an OPG. Axial T2 images (*A, B*) show T2 prolongation and marked enlargement of the intraorbital optic nerves, prechiasmatic optic nerves, optic chiasm, and optic tracts. The tumor also involves the cerebral peduncles and midbrain. (*C*) Sagittal 3D T2-SPACE image shows involvement of the hypothalamus, fornices, corpus callosum, tectum, and pons. (*D*) Axial postcontrast T1-SPACE image shows areas of patchy enhancement in the hypothalamus, optic tracts, and right thalamus.

It is important to recognize that a substantial proportion of LGGs are predominantly nonenhancing. One such tumor is the angiocentric glioma (**Fig. 3**), which is hyperintense on T1- and T2-weighted sequences and shows minimal or no enhancement. These tumors are superficial in location and most commonly affect the frontal and temporal lobes.[28]

Molecular aberrations in LGG ultimately converge in abnormal activation of the mitogen-activated

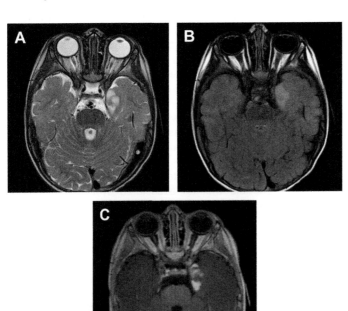

Fig. 2. Ganglioglioma (BRAF V600E positive) in a 14-month-old boy with stereotyped blinking episodes. (*A*) Axial T2 and (*B*) FLAIR images show an expansile lesion with internal T2 prolongation in the left mesial temporal lobe, which shows avid enhancement on (*C*) postcontrast T1-SPACE.

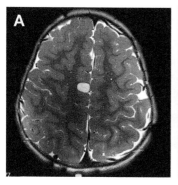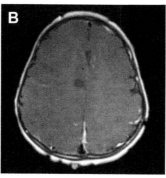

Fig. 3. Angiocentric glioma in a 3-year-old girl presenting with multiple generalized seizures in a single day. (*A*) Axial T2 image shows a well-circumscribed lesion with internal T2 prolongation in the posterior aspect of the right superior frontal lobe. (*B*) Axial T1-SPACE image shows no enhancement.

protein kinase (MAPK) pathway. This pathway starts at the cell membrane with the tyrosine kinase receptor, a transmembrane protein that binds to an extracellular growth factor, resulting in the activation of the intracellular signal transducer RAS. In turn, RAS activates 2 distinct intracellular cascades that activate nuclear transcription factors, which promote cell growth.[29,30] The pathway most frequently affected in LGG is the RAS-BRAF-MAPK extracellular signal-regulated kinase (ERK) pathway.[31] The most common genetic alteration in this pathway is the KIAA1549:BRAF fusion, which is present in 47% of LGGs, including most pilocytic astrocytomas. A second alteration in this pathway is the BRAFV600E point deletion, which occurs in 13% of LGGs, principally in gangliogliomas, PXA, and

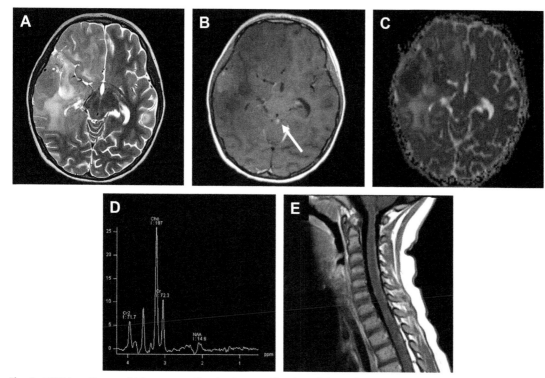

Fig. 4. HGG in a 3-year-old boy presenting in status epilepticus. (*A*) Axial T2 image shows a lesion with intermediate signal in the right superior temporal lobe, with ill-defined T2 prolongation extending into the adjacent white matter. Expansion of the cortex in the right temporal lobe and inferior frontal lobe raises concern for tumor infiltration. (*B*) Axial postcontrast T1-SPACE image shows mild enhancement in the lesion as well as a small focus of leptomeningeal enhancement adjacent to the left superior cerebellar peduncle (*arrow*). (*C*) ADC shows decreased diffusivity in the lesion, which also extends into the right mesial temporal lobe and inferior frontal lobe. (*D*) MRS (TE: 135 milliseconds) shows marked elevation of Cho and marked decrease in NAA, features that indicate a high-grade tumor. (*E*) Sagittal T1 image of the cervical spine shows diffuse leptomeningeal enhancement consistent with tumor dissemination.

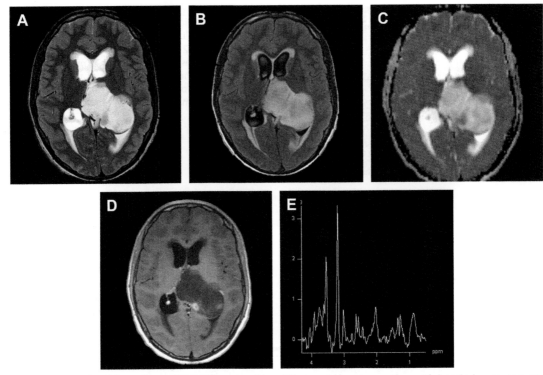

Fig. 5. High-grade midline glioma (H3 K27M mutant) in a 16-year-old boy presenting with headache, nausea, and altered mental status. (*A*) Axial T2 and (*B*) FLAIR images show an expansile lesion centered in the left thalamus with mass effect that results in obstruction of the aqueduct and acute hydrocephalus. (*C*) Axial ADC map shows a small focus of decreased diffusivity that correlates with a nodule of enhancement in the left thalamus on (*D*) post-contrast T1-SPACE. (*E*) MRS (TE: 135 milliseconds) shows elevation of Cho and depletion of NAA.

diffuse gliomas, and in a small percentage of pilocytic astrocytomas (particularly extracerebellar).[32,33] The second pathway associated with MAPK signaling is the phosphoinositide 3 kinase–serine threonine protein kinase–mammalian target of rapamycin (mTOR) pathway. Mutations of regulatory proteins of this pathway also increase predisposition to LGGs. Specifically, patients with NF-1 have decreased function of neurofibromin, which downregulates RAS-dependent activation of this pathway; the lack of inhibition results in the increased risk of LGG seen in up to 20% of NF-1 patients. Similarly, deficiencies in mTOR inhibitors are responsible for the increased risk of LGGs observed in tuberous sclerosis patients.[31]

High-grade gliomas

Although pediatric high-grade gliomas (HGG) represent only 20% of all childhood brain tumors, they account for approximately 44% of brain tumor–related deaths in children less than 14 years of age.[3] The genomics of pediatric HGGs differ substantially from adult HGGs. Approximately 50% of pediatric HGGs harbor mutations involving histone (H) protein complex variants. The remaining HGGs

exhibit a broad variety of mutations that involve other oncogenic pathways, including isocitrate dehydrogenase mutations (<5% of pediatric HGG), several growth factors (eg, platelet-derived growth factor receptor alpha, epithelial growth factor receptor), and the mesenchymal epithelial transition (MET) oncogene. The incidence of pediatric HGGs is also increased in cancer predisposition syndromes, such as Li-Fraumeni and biallelic mismatch repair deficiency.[29]

Hemispheric pediatric HGGs, including glioblastomas, often harbor mutations in the H3.3 variant gene (H3.3G34R/V). These tumors have variable appearance on imaging, but trend toward decreased diffusivity and low signal intensity on T2-weighted sequences, owing to high tumor cellularity (**Fig. 4**). Histologically, there is high vascularity and neovascularity, which manifest as areas of enhancement with elevated CBV.[34] Supratentorial midline HGGs have also been associated with mutations in H3.3. variants. Specifically, H3.3K27M has been reported in a high number of thalamic gliomas.[35] The latter tumors frequently demonstrate T2 prolongation, expansile characteristics, and ill-defined/infiltrating borders. Despite their high grade, less than 50% of thalamic HGGs enhance with contrast (**Fig. 5**).[36]

Posterior Fossa Tumors

Approximately 30% of tumors in children younger than 14 years of age arise in the posterior fossa. In addition, posterior fossa tumors are responsible for slightly more than half of tumor-related deaths in this age group.[3] The most common histologic subtypes observed include MB, ependymoma, and cerebellar juvenile pilocytic astrocytoma (JPA).

Medulloblastoma

MB is the most common posterior fossa tumor of childhood, accounting for approximately one-third of lesions in this location and 9.3% of all tumors in children less than 14 years of age.[3,37] These highly aggressive embryonal tumors are responsible for 14.3% of brain tumor–related deaths in children, second to high-grade glial tumors.[3]

MBs appear as hyperdense, heterogeneous masses on CT. On MR imaging, the tumor demonstrates relatively low signal on T2-weighted sequences and decreased diffusivity. Cystic components, calcification, and rarely, hemorrhage can be seen. After the administration of contrast, MBs show variable enhancement (**Fig. 6**). Perfusion characteristics are also variable, with an overall trend toward elevated CBV.[38] MRS shows elevated Cho as well as Cho/Cr and Cho/NAA ratios. Taurine is a small amino acid that can occasionally be seen in MB, with a resonance frequency of 3.3 ppm. Because of the small size of the molecule, the peak is best appreciated on short TE acquisitions, although it can also be seen on intermediate TE acquisitions as an inverted peak.[39]

For treatment planning, each individual patient is stratified into an average-risk or high-risk group. The stratification incorporates clinical data, imaging data, and CSF analyses. High-risk patients are those younger than 3 years of age, who have CSF dissemination by MR imaging or CSF analysis, or have residual tumor that exceeds 1.5 cm^3 after surgery. To facilitate accurate and timely stratification, spinal MR imaging should be performed before surgery, because postoperative blood products and collections can obscure metastatic deposits. Whenever possible, postoperative imaging to determine residual tumor at the primary site should be performed within the first 2 days after surgery.[40]

The 2007 WHO classification of brain tumors classified MB into 4 categories: classic, large cell/anaplastic, desmoplastic, and MB with extensive nodularity. The 2016 classification incorporates the molecular profile of the tumor and has grouped them into 4 categories: wingless (Wnt), sonic hedgehog (SHH), group 3, and group 4.[41] These designations have important prognostic implications and

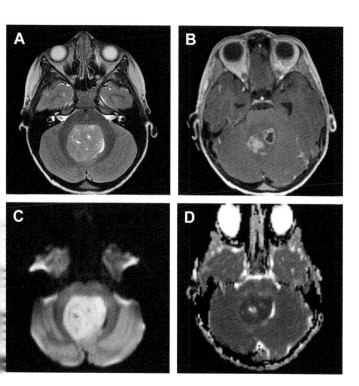

Fig. 6. Group 4 MB in a 5-year-old boy with headaches and altered mental status. (*A*) Axial T2 image shows a mass in the midaspect of the fourth ventricle with low T2 signal intensity. (*B*) Axial postcontrast T1-SPACE shows a predominantly nonenhancing tumor with some areas of nodular rim enhancement. (*C*) Trace diffusion and (*D*) ADC map show markedly decreased diffusivity.

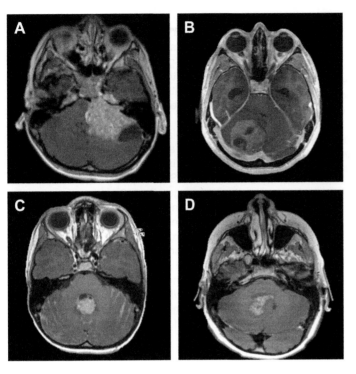

Fig. 7. Imaging phenotype of various groups of MB on postcontrast T1-weighted images. Wnt tumors are located in the cerebellar peduncle (*A*); SHH tumors are centered in the cerebellar hemispheres (*B*); group 3 tumors are located in the midline and show enhancement (*C*); and group 4 tumors are located in the midline and are commonly nonenhancing (*D*). Note that in panel (*C*), the group 3 tumor shows leptomeningeal dissemination in the cerebellar folia (at presentation).

clinical associations. For instance, group 3 tumors have the worst prognosis, followed by group 4; SHH MBs have an intermediate prognosis, and Wnt MBs have a favorable prognosis.[39,41] Imaging correlates to these genomic groups also have been identified (**Fig. 7**).[42] **Table 2** provides details on clinical and imaging associations of MB molecular subtypes.[42,43] Preliminary evidence suggests group-specific spectral patterns, with high taurine peak and low levels of lipids in group 3 and 4 MBs, and high Cho and lipid peaks in SHH MBs

with only trace or absent taurine.[44] Recently, machine learning approaches have proven useful in correctly discriminating among various groups of MB.[45] It is likely that these approaches will become widespread for additional brain tumors in the near future.

Ependymoma

Ependymomas constitute approximately 5.3% of brain tumors in children younger than 14 years of age, with a peak incidence in children younger

Table 2
Imaging and clinical correlates of molecular subgroups in medulloblastoma

Feature	Wnt	SHH	Group 3	Group 4
Approximate frequency, %	10	30	20	40
Location of primary tumor	Cerebellopontine angle	Cerebellar hemisphere (off midline)	Fourth ventricle (midline)	Fourth ventricle (midline)
Enhancement	Variable	Avid enhancement	Common	Predominantly nonenhancing
Appearance of metastasis	Rarely metastatic	Rarely metastatic When observed: nodular and in the posterior fossa	Laminar (almost exclusively)	Nodular (more frequent) Laminar (occasional) Involvement of the anterior third ventricle

Data from Perreault S, Ramaswamy V, Achrol AS, et al. MRI surrogates for molecular subgroups of medulloblastoma. AJNR Am J Neuroradiol 2014;35(7):1263–9; and Zapotocky M, Mata-Mbemba D, Sumerauer D, et al. Differential patterns of metastatic dissemination across medulloblastoma subgroups. J Neurosurg Pediatr 2018;21(2):145–52.

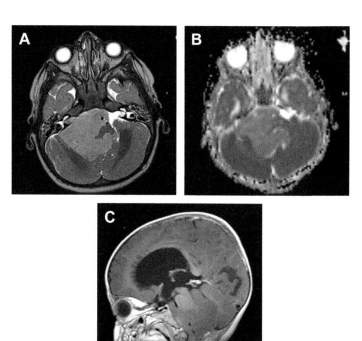

Fig. 8. Posterior fossa ependymoma (group A) in a 15-month-old infant with an enlarging head circumference. (A) Axial T2 image shows a fourth ventricular tumor that extends through the right (greater than left) foramina of Luschka, involves the pontine cistern, invades the right internal auditory canal, and encases the basilar artery. (B) Axial ADC through the lesion shows that the tumor has mildly facilitated diffusion relative to the cerebellar parenchyma. (C) Sagittal postcontrast T1-SPACE image shows nonenhancing tumor that insinuates itself along the CSF spaces of the posterior fossa.

than 5 years. Approximately two-thirds of ependymomas occur in the posterior fossa.[3]

On imaging, ependymomas have a heterogeneous appearance owing to a variety of morphologic features, including solid components, cystic components, hemorrhage, necrosis, and calcification. Calcifications occur more frequently in ependymomas than in other posterior fossa

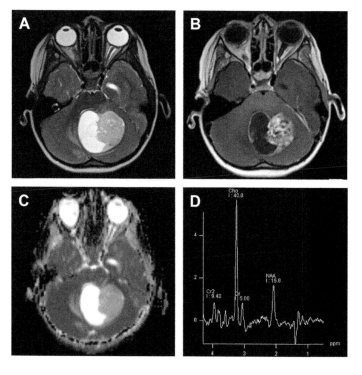

Fig. 9. Pilocytic astrocytoma in a 7-year-old boy with worsening headaches. (A) Axial T2 image shows a mass in the posterior fossa with cystic and solid components. (B) Axial postcontrast T1-SPACE image shows avid enhancement of the solid nodular component of the mass. (C) ADC shows increased diffusivity relative to the brain parenchyma. (D) MRS (TE: 135 milliseconds) shows an elevated Cho peak, a feature that can often be observed in pilocytic astrocytomas despite their low-grade nature.

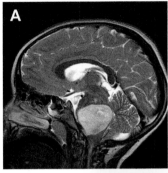
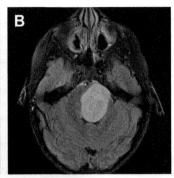
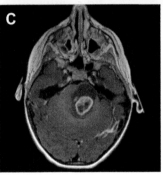

Fig. 10. High-grade midline glioma of the pons in a 4-year-old girl with abnormal eye movements and unsteady gait. (*A*) Sagittal T2 and (*B*) axial FLAIR images show a markedly expansile lesion with internal T2 prolongation in the pons. (*C*) Axial postcontrast T1-SPACE shows ring enhancement, likely necrosis, within the nonenhancing tumor.

tumors. On MR imaging, ependymomas demonstrate low signal on T1-weighted images, intermediate to high signal on T2-weighted images, and moderately decreased diffusivity, which can overlap with that of MB (**Fig. 8**). Contrast enhancement is variable; many tumors demonstrate avid enhancement, whereas others are predominantly nonenhancing.[39] Perfusion MR imaging usually demonstrates moderately elevated CBV as well as high permeability. MRS contributes to the diagnosis by showing elevated myoinositol.[46] The primary location of the tumor provides some specificity to the imaging appearance; most tumors arise in the floor of the fourth ventricle, near the obex, or in the lateral recesses near the foramina of Luschka. Ependymomas spread through the foramina of Luschka and Magendie early in the course of disease.[47]

Ependymomas in the posterior fossa are classified into 2 different molecular subgroups, ependymoma A and ependymoma B. Ependymoma A constitutes the predominant subtype at 80%, characterized by a positive CPG island methylated phenotype (CIMP) that results in trimethylation of H3K27 and dysregulation of gene expression.[48] This subgroup affects infants and young children less than the age of 5 years, with poor prognosis. Conversely, ependymoma B has a CIMP-negative phenotype, affects older children and adolescents, and has a better prognosis. It should be noted that posterior fossa ependymomas are

molecularly distinct from supratentorial and spinal ependymomas.

Juvenile pilocytic astrocytoma
JPA constitutes approximately 35% of all posterior fossa tumors. As previously mentioned, more than half of JPAs occur in the posterior fossa (40% in the cerebellar hemispheres and 20% in the brainstem).[39] For a more detailed discussion of JPA genomics, please see the section on LGG. The classic appearance of these tumors is that of a cystic lesion with an avidly enhancing mural nodule (**Fig. 9**).[39]

Brainstem gliomas
Brainstem gliomas are a heterogeneous group of tumors that includes LGGs and HGGs. LGGs in the brainstem show indolent growth, with good prognosis. These lesions are treated conservatively because of the morbidity of treatment.[21] The role of the radiologist is to ensure stability across serial examinations and identify complications related to increasing mass effect, hydrocephalus, or enlarging cystic components.[49] Common histologic subtypes of LGGs in the brainstem include pilocytic and pilomyxoid astrocytomas.

Most brainstem HGGs are part of the diffuse midline glioma subgroup. Like supratentorial HGGs, these tumors have histone variant mutations. H3-K27M is the most common genotype observed in posterior fossa HGGs and has been described in tumors involving the pons, cerebellar vermis, and upper cervical cord. The most common genotypes of these tumors involve mutations in the H3.1 and H3.3 histone complex proteins. Recent genomic analyses suggest that these 2 tumor populations have distinct biologic behaviors; tumors harboring H3.3 mutations show less sensitivity to radiotherapy, earlier relapse after treatment, and higher risk of distant metastases.[35]

On MR imaging, posterior fossa HGGs show marked expansion of the pons, infiltrative T2 prolongation, and absent or minimal enhancement. The enlargement of the pons may result in complete effacement of the prepontine cistern, and rarely, encasement of the basilar artery by tumor.[39] Focal areas of decreased diffusivity can occasionally be seen, indicating regions of high cellularity (**Fig. 10**).[39] Quantitative analyses also show that apparent diffusion coefficient (ADC) values and histogram metrics are helpful prognostic markers of progression-free survival.[50] Although MRS in the posterior fossa is technically challenging owing to proximity of the osseous skull base, it can help differentiate these tumors from lower-grade neoplasms that show comparatively lower Cho, Cho/Cr, and Cho/NAA.[19,39] MRS can also be used to evaluate response to radiotherapy, with a decrease in lactate and lipid peaks indicating good response.[51]

SUMMARY

Brain tumors are an important cause of morbidly and mortality in children. Imaging plays a central role in the diagnosis, treatment planning, and follow-up of affected patients. Recent advances in genomics and cancer biology are reshaping the role of imaging leading to further work in radiogenomics and artificial intelligence. Understanding the association between imaging phenotype and tumor genetics as well as the implications related to targeted therapy is increasingly important, given the rapidly evolving molecular landscape of pediatric brain tumors.

REFERENCES

1. Ostrom QT, Gittleman H, Truitt G, et al. CBTRUS statistical report: primary brain and other central nervous system tumors diagnosed in the United States in 2011-2015. Neuro Oncol 2018;20(suppl_4):iv1–86.
2. Ostrom QT, Gittleman H, de Blank PM, et al. American Brain Tumor Association adolescent and young adult primary brain and central nervous system tumors diagnosed in the United States in 2008-2012. Neuro Oncol 2016;18(Suppl 1):i1–50.
3. Ostrom QT, de Blank PM, Kruchko C, et al. Alex's Lemonade Stand Foundation infant and childhood primary brain and central nervous system tumors diagnosed in the United States in 2007-2011. Neuro Oncol 2015;16(Suppl 10):x1–36.
4. Hukin J, Siffert J, Cohen H, et al. Leptomeningeal dissemination at diagnosis of pediatric low-grade neuroepithelial tumors. Neuro Oncol 2003;5(3):188–96.
5. Jaspan T, Morgan PS, Warmuth-Metz M, et al. Response assessment in pediatric neuro-oncology: implementation and expansion of the RANO criteria in a randomized phase II trial of pediatric patients with newly diagnosed high-grade gliomas. AJNR Am J Neuroradiol 2016;37(9):1581–7.
6. Warren KE, Vezina G, Poussaint TY, et al. Response assessment in medulloblastoma and leptomeningeal seeding tumors: recommendations from the Response Assessment in Pediatric Neuro-Oncology Committee. Neuro Oncol 2018;20(1):13–23.
7. Warren KE, Poussaint TY, Vezina G, et al. Challenges with defining response to antitumor agents in pediatric neuro-oncology: a report from the Response Assessment in Pediatric Neuro-Oncology (RAPNO) working group. Pediatr Blood Cancer 2013;60(9):1397–401.
8. Higano S, Takahashi S, Kurihara N, et al. Supratentorial primary intra-axial tumors in children. MR and CT evaluation. Acta Radiol 1997;38(6):945–52.
9. Robertson RL, Silk S, Ecklund K, et al. Imaging optimization in children. J Am Coll Radiol 2018;15(3 Pt A):440–3.
10. Ngo AV, Winant AJ, Lee EY, et al. Strategies for reducing radiation dose in CT for pediatric patients: how we do it. Semin Roentgenol 2018;53(2):124–31.
11. Jeevanandham B, Kalyanpur T, Gupta P, et al. Comparison of post-contrast 3D-T1-MPRAGE, 3D-T1-SPACE and 3D-T2-FLAIR MR images in evaluation of meningeal abnormalities at 3-T MRI. Br J Radiol 2017;90(1074):20160834.
12. Poussaint TY, Siffert J, Barnes PD, et al. Hemorrhagic vasculopathy after treatment of central nervous system neoplasia in childhood: diagnosis and follow-up. AJNR Am J Neuroradiol 1995;16(4):693–9.
13. Mikami T, Minamida Y, Yamaki T, et al. Cranial nerve assessment in posterior fossa tumors with fast imaging employing steady-state acquisition (FIESTA). Neurosurg Rev 2005;28(4):261–6.
14. Buch K, Caruso P, Ebb D, et al. Balanced steady-state free precession sequence (CISS/FIESTA/3D Driven Equilibrium Radiofrequency Reset Pulse) increases the diagnostic yield for spinal drop metastases in children with brain tumors. AJNR Am J Neuroradiol 2018;39(7):1355–61.
15. Hayes LL, Jones RA, Palasis S, et al. Drop metastases to the pediatric spine revealed with diffusion-weighted MR imaging. Pediatr Radiol 2012;42(8):1009–13.

16. Welker K, Boxerman J, Kalnin A, et al. ASFNR recommendations for clinical performance of MR dynamic susceptibility contrast perfusion imaging of the brain. AJNR Am J Neuroradiol 2015;36(6): E41–51.

17. O'Connor JP, Jackson A, Parker GJ, et al. DCE-MRI biomarkers in the clinical evaluation of antiangiogenic and vascular disrupting agents. Br J Cancer 2007;96(2):189–95.

18. Grade M, Hernandez Tamames JA, Pizzini FB, et al. A neuroradiologist's guide to arterial spin labeling MRI in clinical practice. Neuroradiology 2015; 57(12):1181–202.

19. Brandao LA, Poussaint TY. Pediatric brain tumors. Neuroimaging Clin N Am 2013;23(3):499–525.

20. Oz G, Alger JR, Barker PB, et al. Clinical proton MR spectroscopy in central nervous system disorders. Radiology 2014;270(3):658–79.

21. Chalil A, Ramaswamy V. Low grade gliomas in children. J Child Neurol 2016;31(4):517–22.

22. Sievert AJ, Fisher MJ. Pediatric low-grade gliomas. J Child Neurol 2009;24(11):1397–408.

23. Koeller KK, Rushing EJ. From the archives of the AFIP: pilocytic astrocytoma: radiologic-pathologic correlation. Radiographics 2004;24(6):1693–708.

24. de Fatima Vasco Aragao M, Law M, Batista de Almeida D, et al. Comparison of perfusion, diffusion, and MR spectroscopy between low-grade enhancing pilocytic astrocytomas and high-grade astrocytomas. AJNR Am J Neuroradiol 2014;35(8):1495–502.

25. Seeburg DP, Dremmen MH, Huisman TA. Imaging of the sella and parasellar region in the pediatric population. Neuroimaging Clin N Am 2017;27(1):99–121.

26. Moore W, Mathis D, Gargan L, et al. Pleomorphic xanthoastrocytoma of childhood: MR imaging and diffusion MR imaging features. AJNR Am J Neuroradiol 2014;35(11):2192–6.

27. Luyken C, Blumcke I, Fimmers R, et al. Supratentorial gangliogliomas: histopathologic grading and tumor recurrence in 184 patients with a median follow-up of 8 years. Cancer 2004;101(1):146–55.

28. Ni HC, Chen SY, Chen L, et al. Angiocentric glioma: a report of nine new cases, including four with atypical histological features. Neuropathol Appl Neurobiol 2015;41(3):333–46.

29. AlRayahi J, Zapotocky M, Ramaswamy V, et al. Pediatric brain tumor genetics: what radiologists need to know. Radiographics 2018;38(7):2102–22.

30. Pakneshan S, Salajegheh A, Smith RA, et al. Clinicopathological relevance of BRAF mutations in human cancer. Pathology 2013;45(4):346–56.

31. Gajjar A, Pfister SM, Taylor MD, et al. Molecular insights into pediatric brain tumors have the potential to transform therapy. Clin Cancer Res 2014;20(22): 5630–40.

32. Schindler G, Capper D, Meyer J, et al. Analysis of BRAF V600E mutation in 1,320 nervous system tumors reveals high mutation frequencies in pleomorphic xanthoastrocytoma, ganglioglioma and extra-cerebellar pilocytic astrocytoma. Acta Neuropathol 2011;121(3):397–405.

33. Jones DT, Kocialkowski S, Liu L, et al. Tandem duplication producing a novel oncogenic BRAF fusion gene defines the majority of pilocytic astrocytomas. Cancer Res 2008;68(21):8673–7.

34. Chang YW, Yoon HK, Shin HJ, et al. MR imaging of glioblastoma in children: usefulness of diffusion/perfusion-weighted MRI and MR spectroscopy. Pediatr Radiol 2003;33(12):836–42.

35. Castel D, Philippe C, Calmon R, et al. Histone H3F3A and HIST1H3B K27M mutations define two subgroups of diffuse intrinsic pontine gliomas with different prognosis and phenotypes. Acta Neuropathol 2015;130(6):815–27.

36. Aboian MS, Solomon DA, Felton E, et al. Imaging characteristics of pediatric diffuse midline gliomas with histone H3 K27M mutation. AJNR Am J Neuroradiol 2017;38(4):795–800.

37. Ostrom QT, Gittleman H, Liao P, et al. CBTRUS statistical report: primary brain and other central nervous system tumors diagnosed in the United States in 2010-2014. Neuro Oncol 2017;19(suppl_5) :v1–88.

38. Yeom KW, Mitchell LA, Lober RM, et al. Arterial spin-labeled perfusion of pediatric brain tumors. AJNR Am J Neuroradiol 2014;35(2):395–401.

39. Brandao LA, Young Poussaint T. Posterior fossa tumors. Neuroimaging Clin N Am 2017;27(1):1–37.

40. Rutkowski S, von Hoff K, Emser A, et al. Survival and prognostic factors of early childhood medulloblastoma: an international meta-analysis. J Clin Oncol 2010;28(33):4961–8.

41. Taylor MD, Northcott PA, Korshunov A, et al. Molecular subgroups of medulloblastoma: the current consensus. Acta Neuropathol 2012;123(4):465–72.

42. Perreault S, Ramaswamy V, Achrol AS, et al. MRI surrogates for molecular subgroups of medulloblastoma. AJNR Am J Neuroradiol 2014;35(7): 1263–9.

43. Zapotocky M, Mata-Mbemba D, Sumerauer D, et al. Differential patterns of metastatic dissemination across medulloblastoma subgroups. J Neurosurg Pediatr 2018;21(2):145–52.

44. Bluml S, Margol AS, Sposto R, et al. Molecular subgroups of medulloblastoma identification using noninvasive magnetic resonance spectroscopy. Neuro Oncol 2016;18(1):126–31.

45. Iv M, Zhou M, Shpanskaya K, et al. MR imaging-based radiomic signatures of distinct molecular subgroups of medulloblastoma. AJNR Am J Neuroradiol 2019;40(1):154–61.

46. Schneider JF, Confort-Gouny S, Viola A, et al. Multiparametric differentiation of posterior fossa tumors in children using diffusion-weighted imaging and

short echo-time 1H-MR spectroscopy. J Magn Reson Imaging 2007;26(6):1390–8.

47. Raybaud C, Ramaswamy V, Taylor MD, et al. Posterior fossa tumors in children: developmental anatomy and diagnostic imaging. Childs Nerv Syst 2015;31(10):1661–76.

48. Mack SC, Witt H, Piro RM, et al. Epigenomic alterations define lethal CIMP-positive ependymomas of infancy. Nature 2014;506(7489): 445–50.

49. Ahmed KA, Laack NN, Eckel LJ, et al. Histologically proven, low-grade brainstem gliomas in children: 30-year experience with long-term follow-up at Mayo Clinic. Am J Clin Oncol 2014;37(1):51–6.

50. Poussaint TY, Vajapeyam S, Ricci KI, et al. Apparent diffusion coefficient histogram metrics correlate with survival in diffuse intrinsic pontine glioma: a report from the Pediatric Brain Tumor Consortium. Neuro Oncol 2016;18(5):725–34.

51. Laprie A, Pirzkall A, Haas-Kogan DA, et al. Longitudinal multivoxel MR spectroscopy study of pediatric diffuse brainstem gliomas treated with radiotherapy. Int J Radiat Oncol Biol Phys 2005; 62(1):20–31.

MR Perfusion and MR Spectroscopy of Brain Neoplasms

Karem Gharzeddine, MD[a], Vaios Hatzoglou, MD[b], Andrei I. Holodny, MD[c],*, Robert J. Young, MD[d]

KEYWORDS

- MR imaging • Perfusion • Spectroscopy • Brain neoplasms

KEY POINTS

- MR perfusion has become a mainstay in the early and prompt characterization of treated lesions, distinguishing inflammatory/reactive processes from actual treatment failure and disease progression.
- MR spectroscopy's ability to interrogate the molecular composition of tumors (eg, 2-hydroxyglutarate) is promising to allow noninvasive diagnosis and guide treatment with molecular targeting methods.
- MR Perfusion and spectroscopy also play a problem solving role in indeterminate tumors with uncertain behavior; identifying higher grade components (and guiding biopsies), monitoring low grade tumors for signs of transformation and early detection of high grade recurrent foci.

MR PERFUSION

Techniques and Imaging Protocols

Three major techniques have been used to perform perfusion-weighted imaging: (1) dynamic susceptibility contrast (DSC), (2) dynamic contrast enhancement (DCE), and (3) arterial spin labeling. These differ in the labeling method, type of images acquired, and parameters measured. Therefore, each method has different advantages and disadvantages. In brief, DSC uses susceptibility imaging, T2*, to detect loss of signal caused by the paramagnetic contrast material. This technique is fast and robust, taking advantage of first-pass imaging and magnification of the contrast-induced signal loss through the susceptibility weighting of images. However, this technique may be limited by susceptibility artifacts from blood, calcifications, foreign/surgical material, and large vessels. Contrast preloading, and gamma variate curve fitting, are commonly used to reduce T1 and leakage effects.

DCE is a T1-weighted sequence that has the advantages of higher spatial resolution than DSC and is less prone to susceptibility artifacts. However, these advantages come at the expense of longer acquisition times and more complex pharmacokinetic modeling, which are reliant on the arterial input function selection.

Arterial spin labeling is the only perfusion method that does not use contrast agents and therefore is advantageous in certain patient populations, such as children. However, this technique is limited by low signal to noise ratio and limited spatial resolution. Increasing the acquisition time is often necessary to overcome these issues.

Dr R.J. Young has received support from NordicNeuroLab, Agios, Puma, and ICON. The remaining authors have nothing to disclose.

[a] Department of Radiology, Memorial Sloan-Kettering Cancer Center, 1275 York Avenue, New York, NY 10065, USA; [b] Department of Radiology, Memorial Sloan-Kettering Cancer Center, Weill Medical College of Cornell University, 1275 York Avenue, New York, NY 10065, USA; [c] Department of Radiology, Memorial Sloan-Kettering Cancer Center, Weill Medical College of Cornell University, Weill Cornell Graduate School of Medical Sciences, 1275 York Avenue, New York, NY 10065, USA; [d] Brain Imaging, Neuroradiology Research, Neuroradiology Service, Department of Radiology, Memorial Sloan Kettering Cancer Center, 1275 York Avenue, New York, NY 10065, USA
* Corresponding author.
E-mail address: holodnya@mskcc.org

Radiol Clin N Am 57 (2019) 1177–1188
https://doi.org/10.1016/j.rcl.2019.07.008

radiologic.theclinics.com

Table 1
T1 DCE MR imaging brain protocol example

Series Description	AX, T1 DCE, PERF	AX, T1 DCE, PERF	AX, T1 DCE, PERF	AX, T1 DCE, PERF
Scanner, examination	3-T brain	3-T brain	1.5-T brain	1.5-T brain
Acquisition sequence	DISCO	SPGR	DISCO	SPGR
Coverage	Brain	Brain (28–32 LOCS)	Brain	Brain
Fat suppression	None	None	None	None
Slice thickness, mm	5	5	5	5
Number of locs/slices	30–36	28–32	30–36	30–36
Phase temp. res, s	3–4	4–5	3–4	4–5
NEX	0.5–1	0.5–1	0.5–1	0.5
ACCEL. Factor	None	1–2	None	1–2
injection delay	10 phases	10 phases	10 phases	10 phases
FOV, cm	24	25.6	24	25.6
FOV phase /frequency, %	0.8–1	0.8–1	0.8–1	0.8–1
Matrix	224 x 224	256 x 120	196 x 196	128 x 128
Phases n	60	60	60	60
Mask file	Not needed for post-processing	n/a	Not needed for post-processing	n/a
TE	Minimum	Minimum	Minimum	Minimum
Scan duration	Minimum 180 s	Minimum 180 s	Minimum 180 s	Minimum 180 s
Series to send for post-processing	Without sat suppression	Without sat suppression	Without sat suppression	Without sat suppression

Abbreviations: ACCEL, acceleration factor; AX, axial; DISCO, differential subsampling with cartesian ordering; FOV, field of view; LOCS, slices; NEX, number of excitations; n/a, not applicable; PERF, perfusion; SPGR, spoiled gradient recall.

An example of DSC and DCE protocols are presented in **Tables 1** and **2**.[1]

Indications

Treatment of most brain tumors includes surgery, radiation therapy (XRT), and chemotherapy. Treatment-related changes represent a spectrum of nontumoral effects that may mimic tumoral worsening on imaging, despite their disparate underlying histopathologic processes. XRT causes endothelial injury, vascular dilatation, necrosis, and inflammatory disruption of the blood-brain barrier[2] resulting in increased enhancement following contrast administration. The etiologies of contrast enhancement in progressive disease (PD) include neoangiogenesis, vascular proliferation in response to increased blood, oxygen, and nutrient requirements by actively growing tumor.

Evaluation of Pseudoprogression

The most impactful and clinically relevant use of MR perfusion (MRP) has been to differentiate true tumor progression (PD) from pseudoprogression. Advances in treatment of glioblastoma with temozolomide (TMZ) as an adjuvant to XRT have resulted in increased progression-free and overall survival.[3] One of the challenges imposed by this and similar treatments is pseudoprogression, the transient increase in the size of enhancing lesions or new enhancing lesions caused by inflammation and necrosis that can mimic disease progression. Traditionally, the only way to differentiate the two entities required histopathology or clinical and imaging follow-up. The incidence of pseudoprogression is 20% to 30%, and the process characteristically improves or stabilizes spontaneously, without any new treatment. MGMT promoter methylation (hypermethylation of the O^6-methylguanine-DNA-methyltransferase gene), which results in the inactivation of this suicide DNA repair enzyme that may otherwise counter the chemotherapy and XRT, increases susceptibility to TMZ and therefore predisposes to a higher incidence of pseudoprogression.

Table 2
T2* DSC MR imaging brain protocol example

Series Description	Axial T2* DSC Perfusion Post	Axial T2* DSC Perfusion Post
Scanner, examination	3-T brain	1.5-T brain
Acquisition sequence	GRE	GRE ECHO EPI
Coverage	Brain	Brain
Slice thickness, mm	5	5
TE1 / TE2	30	30
TR	1500	1200
NEX	1	1
Injection delay	20 Phase Inject delay / 30 s	5-s inject delay
FOV, cm	24	22 (0.8)
Additional details	10–15 slices to cover lesion	20 slices and 40 phases
		4mL/s injection rate, 20 mL saline chase

Abbreviations: ECHO, echo; EPI, echo-planar imaging; FOV, field of view; GRE, gradient recall echo; NEX, number of excitations.

PD results in substantially increased perfusion caused by tumor-induced neoangiogenesis, whereas pseudoprogression typically does not, despite both presenting with similarly enhancing lesions. Most (85%) instances of pseudoprogression present in the first 3 months[4] after XRT + TMZ treatment, although it has also been observed at up to 6 months or longer. Differentiating the two is clinically essential and substantially impacts the treatment course. Pseudoprogression signifies cellular death, cystic necrosis, and therefore response to treatment, indicating effectiveness of the current treatment strategy. PD, however, denotes actively growing tumor and worsening disease, implying treatment failure and necessitating a change in treatment strategy.

Conventional MR imaging had limited success in differentiating pseudoprogression from PD. Analysis of multiple parameters on conventional MR imaging found only subependymal enhancement to be indicative of pseudoprogression, although its low sensitivity limited its use clinically.[5] Another study found that a fifth percentile apparent diffusion coefficient had limited ability to distinguish pseudoprogression from PD.[6]

MR Perfusion, Dynamic Contrast Enhancement, and Dynamic Susceptibility Contrast: Ability to Distinguish Pseudoprogression from Progressive Disease

DCE and DSC MRP techniques have been shown to reliably differentiate both entities with volumetric histogram measures and normalized ratios more likely yielding significant objective results. Studies using quantitative assessment of perfusion by DCE[4] revealed that normalized plasma volume (Vp; 90% percentile) less than 3.9 had a sensitivity of 92% and specificity of 85% for pseudoprogression. Another significantly reliable DCE parameter is the mean permeability coefficient (Ktrans mean), with normalized ratio of Ktrans mean greater than 3.6 having 79% specificity and 69% sensitivity for PD.[4] Studies using DSC technique also showed that changes in relative cerebral blood volume (rCBV) over time were significantly different between the two entities.

Evaluation of Radiation Necrosis

MRP has found similar utility and value in the evaluation of delayed, unrelenting radiation injury known as radiation necrosis. Radiation necrosis occurs in about 10% of patients after standard fractionated XRT and chemotherapy[7] and in more than 18% after stereotactic radiosurgery.[8,9] Radiation necrosis is directly related to the size, intensity, and fractionation of the radiation dose.

Management of radiation necrosis differs critically from tumor progression. The latter necessitates change in management to try to achieve or maintain tumor control.[10] The former only requires symptomatic control, which often involves chronic steroid therapy, anti-anti-angiogenic therapy, or surgical management for histopathologic diagnosis/symptom relief.

Both entities present with new or enlarging enhancing lesions on conventional MR imaging. Radiologists have relied on morphologic features, such as corpus callosum involvement, new foci, and subependymal involvement; however, these features overlapped significantly and necessitated monitoring over a follow-up period.[11,12]

DCE MRP has superior accuracy over conventional MR imaging in determining radiation necrosis from progression of disease (**Fig. 1**). Two parameters of DCE MRP were found to be useful: Vp, an indirect measure of vascularity, has a sensitivity of 92% and specificity 77%; Ktrans, a measure of leakiness and permeability, is increased more significantly in tumor progression, although less accurate than Vp, with sensitivity of 87% and specificity of 71%.[13] A combination of both parameters improved specificity to 94%, but sensitivity dropped to 79%.

Fluorodeoxyglucose (FDG) PET computed tomography (CT) has good accuracy in determining radiation injury (specificity 82%) but limited success in correctly identifying true progression (sensitivity 68%).[14] The concomitant use of FDG PET CT and MRP Vp results improved the predictive value of radiation injury (specificity of 88%) without improvement in sensitivity to tumor progression, suggesting that a negative FDG PET CT improves confidence in diagnosing radiation injury.

DSC perfusion shows comparable results; percentage of signal-intensity recovery had a sensitivity of 95.65% and specificity 100%,[15] whereas rCBV had sensitivity of 91.3% and specificity of 72.73%. In another study, a rCBV greater than 2.1 was 100% sensitive and 95.2% specific for recurrent metastasis.[16]

Tumor Grading

Another common application for MRP is in grading of gliomas. Gliomas constitute 30% of central nervous system tumors (80% of malignant ones).[17] The World Health Organization classification of gliomas into low grade (II) and high grade (III and IV) based on histopathologic and molecular characteristics determines prognosis and treatment course.[18]

Low-grade gliomas are usually closely followed up in the absence of symptomatic need for surgery. High-grade gliomas are usually treated aggressively with surgery and chemo XRT. Biopsy is an invasive procedure that carries significant morbidity and is sometimes not feasible in eloquent areas or difficult to access locations. In addition, it is susceptible to inherent sampling error; imager guidance may be useful in targeting areas of highest yield. The continued development of new treatments and molecular therapies means that noninvasive diagnosis will become of increasing value and importance.

MRP can differentiate between low- and high-grade gliomas with high accuracy. The DCE parameter Vp mean has 95% specificity with 90.7% sensitivity (area under the curve [AUC], 0.974).[19] Ktrans also demonstrated good

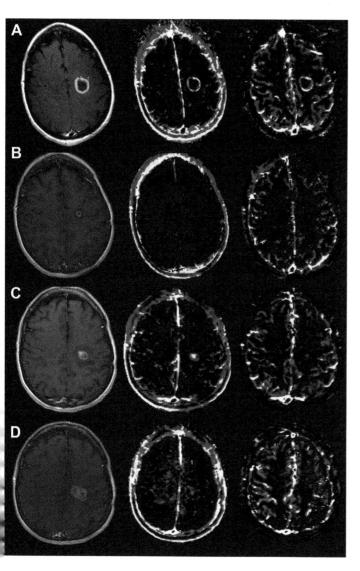

Fig. 1. DCE perfusion MR imaging in a 55-year-old woman with brain metastasis. T1-weighted, Ktrans, and Vp images are shown at multiple time points. (*A*) Pretreatment imaging demonstrates a ring-enhancing lesion with increased permeability constant Ktrans and elevated Vp, indicating viable tumor. (*B–D*) Postradiation treatment follow-up demonstrates initial decrease in tumor size with decreased permeability constant Ktrans and normalization of Vp (*B*) indicating treated disease. Subsequent follow-up, *C* and *D* demonstrate gradual increase in size of the lesion with initial increase in leakiness demonstrated by increased permeability constant Ktrans, seen in inflammation, without appreciable elevation of Vp, a marker of vascular density and viable tumor. In this case, a diagnosis of radiation necrosis was established with higher confidence.

correlation in studies with an accuracy of 91%.[20] The DSC parameter rCBV also correlates well with glioma grade, although with a lower accuracy (AUC, 0.72).[21] Continued improvement in technique, such as histogram analysis,[19] increases objectivity, reliability, and reproducibility.

Oligodendrogliomas are another distinct group of primary brain tumors, comprising 5% to 18% of all gliomas.[22] These tumors are divided into low grade (II) and anaplastic (III) with implications for management and prognosis.[23] The current gold standard for diagnosis is histopathologic analysis following neurosurgical resection. Gross total resection has the possibility of significant morbidity.[24,25] However, subtotal resections or biopsies often have sampling error because of tumor heterogeneity resulting in an accuracy rate in the range of 51% to 83%.[26] MRP shows mixed results

in predicting grade and presence of the 1p/19q codeletion using DSC and DCE techniques. Higher CBV on DSC correlated better with grade than with genetic profile,[27,28] although the accuracy of diagnosis was improved in both compared with conventional MR imaging. Several DCE parameters successfully correlate with tumor grade, including extracellular volume fraction, Ktrans,[29] and Vp.[30] DCE allows quantitative assessment of the entire tumor volume, thus producing more objective and reproducible results.

Response to Treatment in Metastatic Disease

Metastases represent the largest group of intracranial malignancy in adults, constituting up to 40% of brain tumors, with a disease burden of approximately 200,000 cases per year. These are histologically diverse, most commonly lung, breast, genitourinary cancers, osteosarcoma, and melanoma. Advances in radiation treatment, particularly stereotactic radiosurgery, allows for 80% to 90% durable local control.[31] However, a subset of patients fail to respond. Assessment of treatment response noninvasively and promptly has proved challenging by conventional MR imaging size assessment, because up to 50% of treated brain metastases show a transient increase in size, and in a smaller cohort, this increase persists up to 15 months after treatment.[32] In addition, many patients with brain metastases are usually not eligible for surgical treatment and/or biopsy because of advanced systemic disease and poor prognosis. However, early, accurate determination of response/progression remains important to modifying treatment strategies whether for curative or palliative intent. Various studies on MRP, in the immediate post-treatment period (4–12 weeks) have shown consistent results in predicting progression versus treatment response.[33–35]

Tumor Biopsy Guidance

Neurosurgical intervention for biopsy and attempting complete resection carries morbidity and mortality, particularly in inaccessible brain regions and eloquent areas. Additionally, gliomas display a great deal of tumor heterogeneity, resulting in undergrading in 25% of brain tumors when guided by conventional MR imaging[36] and a decreased accuracy of 51% to 83% in another report.[26] MRP provides additional insight into areas with higher vascular concentration (CBV) within enhancing or nonenhancing gliomas and when used to guide the target site, may alter the biopsy targets in up to 54% of cases.[37]

Prognosis

With increased treatment options and improved treatment outcomes, there is an increased need for risk stratification and reliable prognostic factors to manage therapy planning; high-risk patients could be offered additional advanced options at the onset of treatment. In multiple studies, MRP has proven useful in predicting patient prognosis. Both DCE and DSC MRP techniques were found to be accurate predictors of prognosis. rCBV had comparable accuracy to histopathologic World Health Organization grading in mixed gliomas and showed better results in pure astrocytic tumors.[38] Similarly, Ktrans, or vascular leakiness and permeability, and extracellular volume fraction, were inversely correlated with progression-free survival and overall survival.[39]

In primary central nervous system lymphoma, lower perfusion parameters, rCBV in DSC,[40] and Vp and permeability constant Ktrans in DCE[41] were associated with decreased progression-free survival. It is hypothesized that this is possibly caused by decreased vascular density and thus decreased delivery of intravenous chemotherapy and concentration at tumor sites.

Finally, although quantitative assessment, histogram analysis, and normalized ratios are useful to prove superiority in the research setting, a semi-quantitative visual translation of these findings is essential for successful use in the routine clinical setting.

MR SPECTROSCOPY

Whereas conventional MR imaging displays an image reconstruction of anatomic structures and signal intensities, and MRP measures tissue blood flow over time, MR spectroscopy (MRS) interrogates a volume of tissue for its chemical content, which is displayed as a nuclear magnetic resonance spectrum. Specifically, the clinically useful MRS uses the signal from protons bound to methyl groups in the 1- to 5-ppm range of the chemical shift scale. The molecules must be at high enough concentrations to detect, usually in the range of micromoles per gram. The advent of localization techniques allowed interrogation of specific areas and propelled MRS into clinical application. The two widely used clinical techniques are point resolved spectroscopy and stimulated echo acquisition mode.

Metabolites

The number of metabolites that can be resolved on a spectrum is dependent on multiple factors. Besides the metabolite concentration in vivo, the signal to noise ratio is a key factor, which is affected by magnetic field strength and homogeneity and the radiofrequency coil. Additional factors include the specific pulse sequence and imaging parameters, which affect the spectral resolution and therefore determine the number of metabolites that are gleaned.[42,43] Many different molecules have been evaluated for their clinical utility.

- *N*-Acetylaspartate (NAA), a neuronal metabolite with a resonance peak at 2 ppm, has been shown in multiple studies to be exclusively found in neurons and not in glial cells[44–47] and is therefore a marker of neuronal integrity.
- Choline within choline-containing compounds, with a resonance peak at 3.2 ppm, is a constituent of cell membranes and is therefore increased with membrane turnover and cellular proliferation.[48–51]

- Lactate, with a resonance peak at 1.3 ppm, is a marker of anaerobic metabolism and is seen in multiple nontumoral conditions, such as stroke, abscess, and encephalitis. In the setting of a brain tumor, a lactate peak is elevated in necrotic areas, therefore indicating higher grade tumors.[52] Lactate's resonance signal overlaps with that of lipid/macromolecules at 1.3 ppm, but is distinguished by using an intermediate TE, which inverts the lactate signal.
- *Myo*-inositol, with a resonance peak at 3.5 ppm, has been shown to be a marker of gliosis.[53,54]

The role of MRS in brain tumors has been identified since the early 1990s.[55–57] More recent studies have established its utility as an adjunct to conventional MR imaging in improving diagnostic accuracy. Hourani and colleagues[58] demonstrated similar discriminatory capabilities of MRS (accuracy 92%) and perfusion imaging (accuracy 89%) with an improved accuracy of 96% for combining both in differentiating neoplastic and nonneoplastic brain lesions.

In glioma grading, MRS proved superior to conventional imaging alone with an AUC of 0.93 for low- and high-grade tumors (compared with 0.81 and 0.85, respectively, by conventional MR imaging alone).[59] Although MRP was superior in predicting tumor grade, MRS showed some benefit in combination with MRP with a sensitivity of 93% and specificity of 60%.[60] The presence of a lipid/lactate peak associated with necrosis and hypoxia further aids in differentiating higher grade tumors/regions within tumor and correlates with survival[61,62]

Biopsy and Treatment Guidance

In addition to allowing identification of higher grade tumors and higher grade regions within heterogeneous tumor, several studies directly correlated higher choline to NAA levels with cellular density, proliferation index, and cell death index.[63] High choline to NAA ratio (>2) and presence of lactate were more predictive of higher grade tumor (**Fig. 2**).[64] Additional studies demonstrated that incorporating MRS data in the treatment plan, surgery or XRT, aids in tumor delineation, alters treatment, and possibly improves tumor control.[65–67]

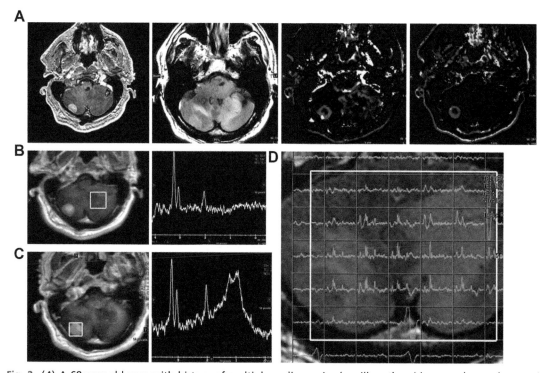

Fig. 2. (*A*) A 68-year-old man with history of multiple malignancies (papillary thyroid cancer, lung adenocarcinoma, and melanoma). DCE perfusion MR imaging revealed a new right cerebellar lesion with increased permeability constant and elevated plasma volume and an expansile pontine/left brachium pontis lesion. (*B*) Single-voxel spectroscopy MRS of the brachium pontis revealed high choline to NAA ratio suggestive of tumor. (*C*) This hyperperfusing right cerebellar tumor was suspected to be either a meningioma or metastasis. (*D*) Multivoxel chemical shift imaging at the same level, demonstrating an MRS pattern more suggestive of metastasis.

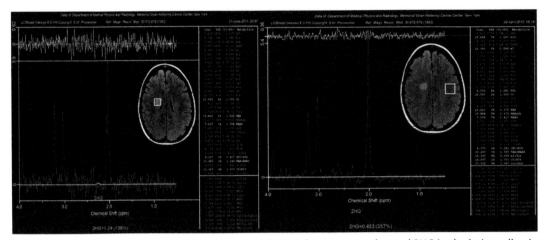

Fig. 3. A 28-year-old woman with incidental lesion. 2HG MRS demonstrates elevated 2HG in the lesion, allowing the diagnosis of a glial tumor based on IDH status noninvasively.

Glioma Versus Solitary Metastasis

Following the same principle, metastases is distinguished from high-grade gliomas by examining the peritumoral edematous areas and normal-looking brain. Glioblastomas tend to have elevated choline/creatine ratio compared with metastases or primary central nervous system lymphoma.[68,69]

MR Spectroscopy, Tumor Stratification, and the Future of Targeted Therapy

The 2016 World Health Organization classification of tumors of the central nervous system update introduced molecular features as criteria of newly defined entities of diffuse gliomas. This has ushered a new era in the approach to diagnosis,

management, and treatment of brain tumors. A noninvasive method to detect surrogate molecules for these genetic alterations is extremely useful, particularly in nonsurgical candidates, to spare or guide biopsies. One such surrogate molecule is 2-hydroxyglutarate (2HG), the direct novel oncometabolite of isocitrate dehydrogenase (IDH) 1 mutated tumors (**Fig. 3**). Most low-grade tumors (about 80%) are IDH mutant. A minority of glioblastomas are also IDH mutant and are thought to represent malignant transformation of lower grade tumors, therefore carrying a better prognosis than IDH-wildtype glioblastoma. Therefore, the ability to make this determination preoperatively aids stratification, prognosis, and treatment planning. New MRS techniques successfully detected 2HG in vivo at 3 T[70,71] in research and clinical

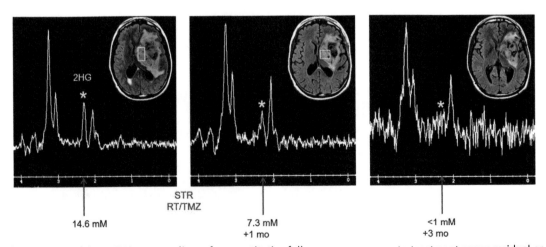

Fig. 4. 2HG peak in an IDH mutant glioma for quantitative follow-up on response to treatment versus residual or recurrent tumor. *, indicates 2hydroxyglutarate peak in the 3 spectra. RT/TMZ, radiation therapy/temozolomide; STR, subtotal resection.

settings.[72] Sensitivity was improved for larger lesions, especially when an idealized 8-mL single voxel could be placed in the lesion. Furthermore, 2HG MRS was shown to be reproducible; predictive of tumor progression, cellularity, and grade; and predictive of response to treatment (Fig. 4).[73] The main challenge of 2HG MRS is limited sensitivity, because the main peak targeted at 2.25 ppm may be admixed with peaks from γ-aminobutyric acid, glutamine, and glutamate. Variable time-to-echo sequences are useful to augment the 2HG signal.

SUMMARY

MRP has become a mainstay in evaluating treatment response and is increasingly important in the diagnostic work-up of primary and metastatic brain disease and determining prognosis. MRS is currently used as a problem-solving technique in diagnosis of brain lesions and assessing post-treatment changes. With increasing knowledge of the molecular basis of tumors and development of molecular targeting therapies, spectroscopy promises to provide a noninvasive method to diagnose tumor types and predict response to new treatment paradigms.

REFERENCES

1. Ellingson BM, Bendszus M, Boxerman J, et al. Consensus recommendations for a standardized brain tumor imaging protocol in clinical trials. Neuro Oncol 2015;17(9):1188–98.
2. Hopewell JW, Calvo W, Jaenke R, et al. Microvasculature and radiation damage. Recent Results Cancer Res 1993;130:1–16.
3. Stupp R, Mason WP, van den Bent MJ, et al. Radiotherapy plus concomitant and adjuvant temozolomide for glioblastoma. N Engl J Med 2005;352(10):987–96.
4. Thomas AA, Arevalo-Perez J, Kaley T, et al. Dynamic contrast enhanced T1 MRI perfusion differentiates pseudoprogression from recurrent glioblastoma. J Neurooncol 2015;125(1):183–90.
5. Young RJ, Gupta A, Shah AD, et al. Potential utility of conventional MRI signs in diagnosing pseudoprogression in glioblastoma. Neurology 2011;76(22):1918–24.
6. Song YS, Choi SH, Park CK, et al. True progression versus pseudoprogression in the treatment of glioblastomas: a comparison study of normalized cerebral blood volume and apparent diffusion coefficient by histogram analysis. Korean J Radiol 2013;14(4):662–72.
7. Ruben JD, Dally M, Bailey M, et al. Cerebral radiation necrosis: incidence, outcomes, and risk factors with emphasis on radiation parameters and chemotherapy. Int J Radiat Oncol Biol Phys 2006;65(2):499–508.
8. Minniti G, Clarke E, Lanzetta G, et al. Stereotactic radiosurgery for brain metastases: analysis of outcome and risk of brain radionecrosis. Radiat Oncol 2011;6:48.
9. Brennan C, Yang TJ, Hilden P, et al. A phase 2 trial of stereotactic radiosurgery boost after surgical resection for brain metastases. Int J Radiat Oncol Biol Phys 2014;88(1):130–6.
10. Field KM, Simes J, Nowak AK, et al. Randomized phase 2 study of carboplatin and bevacizumab in recurrent glioblastoma. Neuro Oncol 2015;17(11):1504–13.
11. Mullins ME, Barest GD, Schaefer PW, et al. Radiation necrosis versus glioma recurrence: conventional MR imaging clues to diagnosis. AJNR Am J Neuroradiol 2005;26(8):1967–72.
12. Rahmathulla G, Marko NF, Weil RJ. Cerebral radiation necrosis: a review of the pathobiology, diagnosis and management considerations. J Clin Neurosci 2013;20(4):485–502.
13. Jahng GH, Li KL, Ostergaard L, et al. Perfusion magnetic resonance imaging: a comprehensive update on principles and techniques. Korean J Radiol 2014;15(5):554–77.
14. Hatzoglou V, Yang TJ, Omuro A, et al. A prospective trial of dynamic contrast-enhanced MRI perfusion and fluorine-18 FDG PET-CT in differentiating brain tumor progression from radiation injury after cranial irradiation. Neuro Oncol 2016;18(6):873–80.
15. Barajas RF, Chang JS, Sneed PK, et al. Distinguishing recurrent intra-axial metastatic tumor from radiation necrosis following gamma knife radiosurgery using dynamic susceptibility-weighted contrast-enhanced perfusion MR imaging. AJNR Am J Neuroradiol 2009;30(2):367–72.
16. Mitsuya K, Nakasu Y, Horiguchi S, et al. Perfusion weighted magnetic resonance imaging to distinguish the recurrence of metastatic brain tumors from radiation necrosis after stereotactic radiosurgery. J Neurooncol 2010;99(1):81–8.
17. Goodenberger ML, Jenkins RB. Genetics of adult glioma. Cancer Genet 2012;205(12):613–21.
18. Louis DN, Perry A, Reifenberger G, et al. The 2016 World Health Organization Classification of Tumors of the Central Nervous System: a summary. Acta Neuropathol 2016;131(6):803–20.
19. Arevalo-Perez J, Peck KK, Young RJ, et al. Dynamic contrast-enhanced perfusion MRI and diffusion-weighted imaging in grading of gliomas. J Neuroimaging 2015;25(5):792–8.
20. Jung SC, Yeom JA, Kim JH, et al. Glioma: application of histogram analysis of pharmacokinetic parameters from T1-weighted dynamic

contrast-enhanced MR imaging to tumor grading. AJNR Am J Neuroradiol 2014;35(6):1103–10.

21. Hilario A, Ramos A, Perez-Nunez A, et al. The added value of apparent diffusion coefficient to cerebral blood volume in the preoperative grading of diffuse gliomas. AJNR Am J Neuroradiol 2012;33(4):701–7.

22. Chawla S, Krejza J, Vossough A, et al. Differentiation between oligodendroglioma genotypes using dynamic susceptibility contrast perfusion-weighted imaging and proton MR spectroscopy. AJNR Am J Neuroradiol 2013;34(8):1542–9.

23. Forst DA, Nahed BV, Loeffler JS, et al. Low-grade gliomas. Oncologist 2014;19(4):403–13.

24. Field M, Witham TF, Flickinger JC, et al. Comprehensive assessment of hemorrhage risks and outcomes after stereotactic brain biopsy. J Neurosurg 2001; 94(4):545–51.

25. Kreth FW, Muacevic A, Medele R, et al. The risk of haemorrhage after image guided stereotactic biopsy of intra-axial brain tumours: a prospective study. Acta Neurochir (Wien) 2001;143(6):539–45 [discussion: 545–6].

26. Pouratian N, Asthagiri A, Jagannathan J, et al. Surgery Insight: the role of surgery in the management of low-grade gliomas. Nat Clin Pract Neurol 2007; 3(11):628–39.

27. Fellah S, Caudal D, De Paula AM, et al. Multimodal MR imaging (diffusion, perfusion, and spectroscopy): is it possible to distinguish oligodendroglial tumor grade and 1p/19q codeletion in the pretherapeutic diagnosis? AJNR Am J Neuroradiol 2013; 34(7):1326–33.

28. Whitmore RG, Krejza J, Kapoor GS, et al. Prediction of oligodendroglial tumor subtype and grade using perfusion weighted magnetic resonance imaging. J Neurosurg 2007;107(3):600–9.

29. Jia Z, Geng D, Liu Y, et al. Low-grade and anaplastic oligodendrogliomas: differences in tumour microvascular permeability evaluated with dynamic contrast-enhanced magnetic resonance imaging. J Clin Neurosci 2013;20(8):1110–3.

30. Arevalo-Perez J, Kebede AA, Peck KK, et al. Dynamic contrast-enhanced MRI in low-grade versus anaplastic oligodendrogliomas. J Neuroimaging 2016;26(3):366–71.

31. Aoyama H, Shirato H, Tago M, et al. Stereotactic radiosurgery plus whole-brain radiation therapy vs stereotactic radiosurgery alone for treatment of brain metastases: a randomized controlled trial. JAMA 2006;295(21):2483–91.

32. Patel TR, McHugh BJ, Bi WL, et al. A comprehensive review of MR imaging changes following radiosurgery to 500 brain metastases. AJNR Am J Neuroradiol 2011;32(10):1885–92.

33. Taunk NK, Oh JH, Shukla-Dave A, et al. Early posttreatment assessment of MRI perfusion biomarkers can predict long-term response of lung cancer brain metastases to stereotactic radiosurgery. Neuro Oncol 2018;20(4):567–75.

34. Almeida-Freitas DB, Pinho MC, Otaduy MC, et al. Assessment of irradiated brain metastases using dynamic contrast-enhanced magnetic resonance imaging. Neuroradiology 2014;56(6):437–43.

35. Jakubovic R, Sahgal A, Soliman H, et al. Magnetic resonance imaging-based tumour perfusion parameters are biomarkers predicting response after radiation to brain metastases. Clin Oncol (R Coll Radiol) 2014;26(11):704–12.

36. Covarrubias DJ, Rosen BR, Lev MH. Dynamic magnetic resonance perfusion imaging of brain tumors. Oncologist 2004;9(5):528–37.

37. Lev MH, Ozsunar Y, Henson JW, et al. Glial tumor grading and outcome prediction using dynamic spin-echo MR susceptibility mapping compared with conventional contrast-enhanced MR: confounding effect of elevated rCBV of oligodendrogliomas [corrected]. AJNR Am J Neuroradiol 2004;25(2):214–21.

38. Spampinato MV, Schiarelli C, Cianfoni A, et al. Correlation between cerebral blood volume measurements by perfusion-weighted magnetic resonance imaging and two-year progression-free survival in gliomas. Neuroradiol J 2013;26(4):385–95.

39. Ulyte A, Katsaros VK, Liouta E, et al. Prognostic value of preoperative dynamic contrast-enhanced MRI perfusion parameters for high-grade glioma patients. Neuroradiology 2016; 58(12):1197–208.

40. Valles FE, Perez-Valles CL, Regalado S, et al. Combined diffusion and perfusion MR imaging as biomarkers of prognosis in immunocompetent patients with primary central nervous system lymphoma. AJNR Am J Neuroradiol 2013;34(1):35–40.

41. Hatzoglou V, Oh JH, Buck O, et al. Pretreatment dynamic contrast-enhanced MRI biomarkers correlate with progression-free survival in primary central nervous system lymphoma. J Neurooncol 2018;140(2):351–8.

42. Gruetter R, Weisdorf SA, Rajanayagan V, et al. Resolution improvements in in vivo 1H NMR spectra with increased magnetic field strength. J Magn Reson 1998;135(1):260–4.

43. Otazo R, Mueller B, Ugurbil K, et al. Signal-to-noise ratio and spectral linewidth improvements between 1.5 and 7 Tesla in proton echo-planar spectroscopic imaging. Magn Reson Med 2006;56(6):1200–10.

44. Urenjak J, Williams SR, Gadian DG, et al. Specific expression of N-acetylaspartate in neurons, oligodendrocyte-type-2 astrocyte progenitors, and immature oligodendrocytes in vitro. J Neurochem 1992;59(1):55–61.

45. Tallan HH. Studies on the distribution of N-acetyl-L-aspartic acid in brain. J Biol Chem 1957;224(1):41–5.

46. Moffett JR, Namboodiri MA, Cangro CB, et al. Immunohistochemical localization of N-acetylaspartate in rat brain. Neuroreport 1991;2(3):131–4.

47. Rigotti DJ, Inglese M, Gonen O. Whole-brain N-acetylaspartate as a surrogate marker of neuronal damage in diffuse neurologic disorders. AJNR Am J Neuroradiol 2007;28(10):1843–9.

48. Howe FA, Barton SJ, Cudlip SA, et al. Metabolic profiles of human brain tumors using quantitative in vivo 1H magnetic resonance spectroscopy. Magn Reson Med 2003;49(2):223–32.

49. Miller BL. A review of chemical issues in 1H NMR spectroscopy: N-acetyl-L-aspartate, creatine and choline. NMR Biomed 1991;4(2):47–52.

50. Licata SC, Renshaw PF. Neurochemistry of drug action: insights from proton magnetic resonance spectroscopic imaging and their relevance to addiction. Ann N Y Acad Sci 2010;1187:148–71.

51. Richards TL. Proton MR spectroscopy in multiple sclerosis: value in establishing diagnosis, monitoring progression, and evaluating therapy. AJR Am J Roentgenol 1991;157(5):1073–8.

52. Al-Okaili RN, Krejza J, Wang S, et al. Advanced MR imaging techniques in the diagnosis of intraaxial brain tumors in adults. Radiographics 2006; 26(Suppl 1):S173–89.

53. Pouwels PJ, Kruse B, Korenke GC, et al. Quantitative proton magnetic resonance spectroscopy of childhood adrenoleukodystrophy. Neuropediatrics 1998;29(5):254–64.

54. Kantarci K, Knopman DS, Dickson DW, et al. Alzheimer disease: postmortem neuropathologic correlates of antemortem 1H MR spectroscopy metabolite measurements. Radiology 2008;248(1): 210–20.

55. Bruhn H, Frahm J, Gyngell ML, et al. Noninvasive differentiation of tumors with use of localized H-1 MR spectroscopy in vivo: initial experience in patients with cerebral tumors. Radiology 1989;172(2): 541–8.

56. Gill SS, Thomas DG, Van Bruggen N, et al. Proton MR spectroscopy of intracranial tumours: in vivo and in vitro studies. J Comput Assist Tomogr 1990; 14(4):497–504.

57. Peeling J, Sutherland G. High-resolution 1H NMR spectroscopy studies of extracts of human cerebral neoplasms. Magn Reson Med 1992;24(1): 123–36.

58. Hourani R, Brant LJ, Rizk T, et al. Can proton MR spectroscopic and perfusion imaging differentiate between neoplastic and nonneoplastic brain lesions in adults? AJNR Am J Neuroradiol 2008;29(2): 366–72.

59. Julia-Sape M, Coronel I, Majos C, et al. Prospective diagnostic performance evaluation of single-voxel 1H MRS for typing and grading of brain tumours. NMR Biomed 2012;25(4):661–73.

60. Law M, Yang S, Wang H, et al. Glioma grading: sensitivity, specificity, and predictive values of perfusion MR imaging and proton MR spectroscopic imaging compared with conventional MR imaging. AJNR Am J Neuroradiol 2003;24(10):1989–98.

61. Murphy PS, Rowland IJ, Viviers L, et al. Could assessment of glioma methylene lipid resonance by in vivo (1)H-MRS be of clinical value? Br J Radiol 2003;76(907):459–63.

62. Crawford FW, Khayal IS, McGue C, et al. Relationship of pre-surgery metabolic and physiological MR imaging parameters to survival for patients with untreated GBM. J Neurooncol 2009;91(3): 337–51.

63. McKnight TR, Lamborn KR, Love TD, et al. Correlation of magnetic resonance spectroscopic and growth characteristics within grades II and III gliomas. J Neurosurg 2007;106(4):660–6.

64. Chang SM, Nelson S, Vandenberg S, et al. Integration of preoperative anatomic and metabolic physiologic imaging of newly diagnosed glioma. J Neurooncol 2009;92(3):401–15.

65. Kallenberg K, Bock HC, Helms G, et al. Untreated glioblastoma multiforme: increased myo-inositol and glutamine levels in the contralateral cerebral hemisphere at proton MR spectroscopy. Radiology 2009;253(3):805–12.

66. Stadlbauer A, Moser E, Gruber S, et al. Improved delineation of brain tumors: an automated method for segmentation based on pathologic changes of 1H-MRSI metabolites in gliomas. Neuroimage 2004;23(2):454–61.

67. Einstein DB, Wessels B, Bangert B, et al. Phase II trial of radiosurgery to magnetic resonance spectroscopy-defined high-risk tumor volumes in patients with glioblastoma multiforme. Int J Radiat Oncol Biol Phys 2012;84(3):668–74.

68. Wijnen JP, Idema AJ, Stawicki M, et al. Quantitative short echo time 1H MRSI of the peripheral edematous region of human brain tumors in the differentiation between glioblastoma, metastasis, and meningioma. J Magn Reson Imaging 2012;36(5): 1072–82.

69. Chawla S, Zhang Y, Wang S, et al. Proton magnetic resonance spectroscopy in differentiating glioblastomas from primary cerebral lymphomas and brain metastases. J Comput Assist Tomogr 2010;34(6): 836–41.

70. Andronesi OC, Kim GS, Gerstner E, et al. Detection of 2-hydroxyglutarate in IDH-mutated glioma patients by in vivo spectral-editing and 2D correlation magnetic resonance spectroscopy. Sci Transl Med 2012;4(116):116ra114.

71. Choi C, Ganji SK, DeBerardinis RJ, et al. 2-hydroxyglutarate detection by magnetic resonance spectroscopy in IDH-mutated patients with gliomas. Nat Med 2012;18(4):624–9.

72. de la Fuente MI, Young RJ, Rubel J, et al. Integration of 2-hydroxyglutarate-proton magnetic resonance spectroscopy into clinical practice for disease monitoring in isocitrate dehydrogenase-mutant glioma. Neuro Oncol 2016;18(2):283–90.

73. Choi C, Raisanen JM, Ganji SK, et al. Prospective longitudinal analysis of 2-hydroxyglutarate magnetic resonance spectroscopy identifies broad clinical utility for the management of patients with IDH-mutant glioma. J Clin Oncol 2016; 34(33):4030–9.

Utility of Preoperative Blood-Oxygen-Level–Dependent Functional MR Imaging in Patients with a Central Nervous System Neoplasm

Ammar A. Chaudhry, MD[a],*, Sohaib Naim, BSc[b], Maryam Gul, MD[b], Abbas Chaudhry, PharmD[b], Mike Chen, MD, PhD[c], Rahul Jandial, MD, PhD[c], Behnam Badie, MD[c]

KEYWORDS

- fMR imaging brain mapping • BOLD fMR imaging • Sensorimotor • Neurovascular uncoupling

KEY POINTS

- Functional MR imaging provides reliable in vivo assessment of the eloquent cortex and can be used to identify sensorimotor, language, and visual regions.
- Key limitations of BOLD task-fMR imaging include:
  - Necessity of patient cooperation and ability of patients to perform the required task, thus limiting its application in young and elderly patients as well as those with neurocognitive limitations.
  - BOLD fMR imaging is motion sensitive.
  - In instances where tumor involves the eloquent cortex, postoperative changes limit BOLD fMR imaging assessment of perisurgical sites.
  - Tumor and tumor microenvironment can affect normal hemodynamic response, resulting in neurovascular uncoupling and leading to false-negative BOLD fMR imaging signal changes.

INTRODUCTION

Functional neuroimaging provides a means to understand the relationship between brain structure and function.[1] Functional MR (fMR) imaging can offer unique insight into preoperative planning for central nervous system (CNS) neoplasms by identifying areas of the brain affected or spared by the neoplasm.[1] The development of fMR imaging presented a breakthrough in imaging acquisition and analysis[1–3] as well as patient management. Since its discovery in 1992 by Ogawa and colleagues, the blood-oxygen-level–dependent (BOLD) fMR imaging technique has become the dominant in vivo imaging technique for functional brain imaging. BOLD fMR imaging provides functional information without requiring invasive electrodes, radiation, or intravenous

Disclosure Statement: The authors have nothing to disclose.
[a] Precision Imaging Lab, Department of Diagnostic Radiology, City of Hope National Cancer Center, 1500 East Duarte Road, Los Angeles, CA 91010, USA; [b] Department of Diagnostic Radiology, City of Hope National Cancer Center, 1500 East Duarte Road, Los Angeles, CA 91010, USA; [c] Department of Neurosurgery, City of Hope National Cancer Center, 1500 East Duarte Road, Los Angeles, CA 91010, USA
* Corresponding author.
E-mail address: achaudhry@coh.org

contrast agent.[1,3–5] The BOLD sequence uses differences in tissue magnetic susceptibility properties (T2* effect) between oxyhemoglobin (diamagnetic) and deoxyhemoglobin (paramagnetic).[1,3,4,6] The BOLD fMR imaging signal depends on cerebral blood flow, cerebral blood volume, and cerebral metabolic rate. The net difference between tissue oxyhemoglobin and deoxyhemoglobin during the hemodynamic response (known as the hemodynamic response function [HRF]) is what generates the MR imaging signal. The "BOLD effect" assesses coupling of oxygenated blood flow and neuronal metabolism during functional tasks, resulting in a net difference in oxyhemoglobin and deoxyhemoglobin, which generates the BOLD signal.[3,4,6] Hemoglobin's magnetic properties depend on the reduction-oxidation of iron between Fe^{2+} and Fe^{3+} states (ie, oxygenated and deoxygenated states). These changes result in an increase in local tissue-derived signal intensity on T2*-weighted MR images.[3–7] BOLD fMR imaging provides good spatial resolution for effective mapping of CNS function in patients whose tumor and/or peritumoral edema is adjacent to eloquent cortex.

This article discusses the applications, significance, and interpretation of BOLD fMR imaging and its relevance to presurgical planning in patients with CNS neoplasms.

BLOOD-OXYGEN-LEVEL–DEPENDENT FUNCTIONAL MR IMAGING AND THE ELOQUENT CORTEX
Sensorimotor

At many medical centers in the United States, BOLD fMR imaging is used to evaluate the sensorimotor system by providing an effective, low-risk, noninvasive means of evaluating the eloquent cortex, comparable with intraoperative mapping techniques.[8] BOLD fMR imaging can be used to identify critical areas of interest to the neurosurgeon by discerning key functional areas of gray matter on structural MR imaging. This is particularly important in settings where tumor and/or peritumoral edema is in close proximity to eloquent cortex. The primary motor cortex, located in the precentral gyrus, is responsible for generating neural impulses that control motor movement. Any significant injury to this region can result in irreversible paresis.[1,8,9] The primary sensory cortex is located in the postcentral gyrus.[8] Separated by the central sulcus, the motor and sensory gyri are somatotopically organized.[10]

In the pre-BOLD fMR imaging era and in instances where BOLD fMR imaging is not available, traditional anatomic landmark approaches are used to identify the precentral gyrus and intraoperative electrodes are used to map out the hand-foot motor regions. Traditionally, the "reverse omega sign" is used to identify the hand motor region; however, this is not always reliable to because of anatomic variation and/or distortion of the homunculus by neoplasm or edema. Motor functions activated by the primary somatosensory cortex, such as the planning, execution, and control of specific behavior, is a complex neural process, and delineating neuronal function solely according to anatomic landmarks can be unreliable.[11] In addition, the lack of reliable anatomic landmarks make it difficult to precisely localize the facial motor region on the precentral gyrus.[12] Supported by clinical and neural data, 3 main motor areas (hand, face/lips/tongue, and foot) can be reliably identified on fMR imaging with good agreement between BOLD fMR imaging maps and intraoperative functional mapping.[12,13] The foot motor region is usually located medially along the parasagittal aspect of the precentral gyrus at the level of the interhemispheric fissure (**Figs. 1** and **2**). The direct intraoperative cortical stimulation of this region is complicated by the presence of the adjacent superior sagittal sinus and can be further complicated by the presence of nearby edema, tumor, and/or aberrant vasculature such as a developmental venous anomaly. The 3 main functional areas (face, hand, foot) span the precentral gyrus (lateral to medial) and can be reliably assessed on task-based fMR imaging.[1] It is important that patients with paresis can elicit motor and sensory activation with sensory stimulation of the hand, face, or foot through induced motor signals.[14,15] During an fMR imaging examination, studies have shown paretic patients to induce more head motion as they experience difficulty moving the affected limb, leading to motion artifact and misregistration of BOLD signal.[1]

Also important are secondary motor areas, which when damaged can lead to significant morbidity, thus increasing the importance of precise fMR imaging localization.[1] The secondary areas of the brain of interest for neurosurgical planning include the pre–supplementary motor area (pre-SMA) and the supplementary motor area (SMA).[16] The SMA consists of a posterior SMA, which is most commonly identified adjacent to the precentral sulcus and is normally active during motor tasks (see **Figs. 1** and **2**).[16] The anterior portion of the SMA (**Fig. 3**) is more active during language activation and its borders are less well defined. Recent studies have suggested that the motor region of the SMA is somatotopically arranged.[16] Studies have shown that direct activation of the SMA influences speech, which is

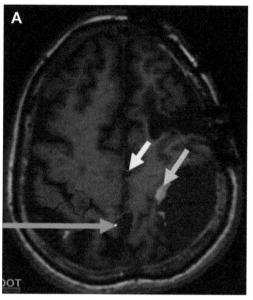
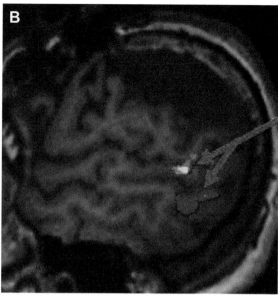

Fig. 1. A 61-year-old woman with recurrent meningioma presented for presurgical evaluation of primary motor cortex. (A) Axial T1-precontrast series depicts recurrent extra-axial dural-based mass along the left posterior cerebral convexity with mass effect on the perirolandic structures. Task-fMR imaging BOLD signal depicts motor activation along the precentral gyrus (left foot, *green arrow*; left hand, *orange arrow*; SMA, *yellow arrow*). (B) Sagittal T1-precontrast images in the same subject depicts Wernicke area (*blue arrows*) along the posterolateral left temporal lobe with variant anatomy.

evident during different language tasks, such as silent verbal fluency and repetition.[17] Motor planning is largely associated with the SMA. Within the SMA is a centralized region that remains active

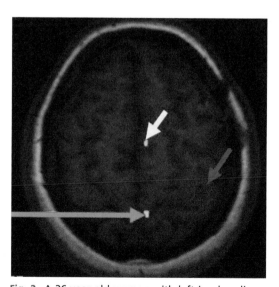

Fig. 2. A 36-year-old woman with left insular glioma presented for preoperative eloquent cortex mapping. Left toe movement elicits activation in the left parasagittal precentral gyrus (*green arrow*), and left finger tap elicits activation along the lateral aspect of the left precentral gyrus (*red arrow*). The SMA is depicted by the yellow arrow.

during both language and motor tasks. It is also acknowledged that the SMA plays an important role in the planning and execution of movements, and that both passive and active tasks can be reliably detected through BOLD fMR imaging.[17]

Because surgical resection of a brain neoplasm poses a risk to the eloquent cortex with potential for permanent neurologic damage, preoperative BOLD fMR imaging is particularly useful in cases where tumor and/or peritumoral edema is in close proximity to eloquent cortex. Using fMR imaging techniques, surgical teams can plan tumor resection through noninvasive visualization of the brain and analysis of lesion localization in relation to anatomic landmarks.[18] Furthermore, fMR imaging derived information can also be used in counseling patients about the risks involved with surgical resection and in prospectively developing an appropriate surgical approach.[19]

Language (Broca and Wernicke Areas) and Memory

The Intracarotid Amobarbital Test, otherwise known as "Wada" testing, has been considered the gold standard for determining the language-dominant hemisphere.[20] Although it is well known that the left cerebral hemisphere is usually the dominant center for language in most of the population, adequate preoperative testing is required to

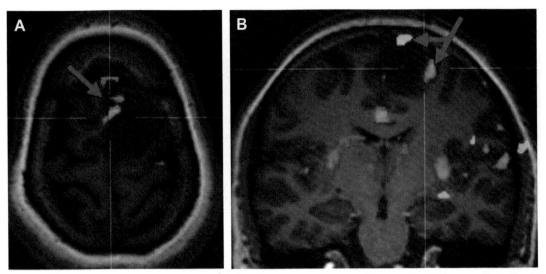

Fig. 3. Axial (*A*) and coronal (*B*) presurgical task-fMR imaging in a 39-year-old woman with history of left frontal oligodendroglioma depicts SMA (*red arrow*) along the anteromedial and lateral margins of the neoplasm, which was confirmed on intraoperative functional mapping.

properly establish cerebral language dominance (**Fig. 4**). Owing to its high level of accuracy in predicting hemispheric language dominance and its noninvasive nature, task-fMR imaging is the standard of care in medical centers where it is available. Silent word-generation paradigms are most commonly used to elicit activation in the Broca area, most commonly located in the inferior frontal gyrus (**Fig. 5**). Silent sentence completion is the most frequently used paradigm to elicit activation in the Wernicke area (see **Fig. 5**). Of importance is that language regions (Wernicke more so than

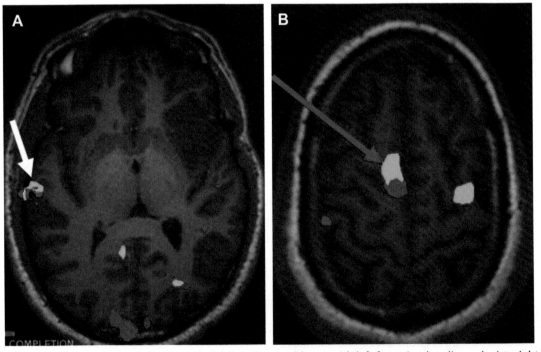

Fig. 4. Preoperative axial task-fMR imaging (*A*) in a 29-year-old man with left frontoinsular glioma depicts right temporal dominance of Wernicke area (*white arrow*). More superiorly, (*B*) there is robust activation of the SMA in the right frontal lobe (*red arrow*).

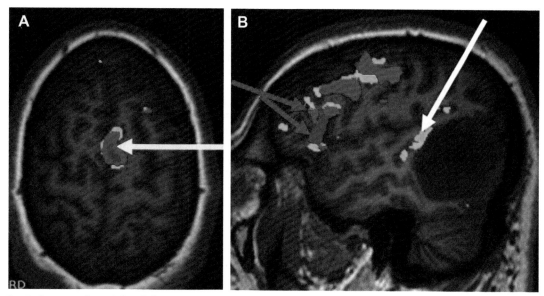

Fig. 5. Preoperative axial task-fMR imaging (*A*) in a 31-year-old man with left temporo-occipital glioma depicts left cerebral language dominance with robust activation of the SMA in the left frontal lobe (*yellow arrow*). Sagittal series (*B*) depicts activation in Broca (*red arrow*) and Wernicke (*white arrow*) regions.

Broca) tend to be somewhat more broadly distributed and require careful image acquisition and postprocessing to ensure accurate depiction of the language network and limit overestimation or underestimation of these regions. To improve precision of localizing Broca and Wernicke regional activity, additional language paradigms are delivered including rhyming, antonym generation, object naming, and/or passive story listening.

Evaluation of memory lateralization is not well established on task-fMR imaging. A case study by Szaflarski and colleagues[21] showed mixed results in the diagnostic accuracy of fMR imaging in predicting the memory outcomes of patients with epilepsy through presurgical evaluation. At present, additional research is required to develop a robust task-fMR or resting-state fMR (rs-fMR) imaging application for memory assessment. Such a development can be applied in the preoperative setting for patients with tumor or epilepsy, but can also be extended to evaluation of neurodegenerative diseases.[10]

PITFALLS OF BLOOD-OXYGEN-LEVEL–DEPENDENT FUNCTIONAL MR IMAGING

During an fMR imaging scan, it is common to find artifacts in patients with brain tumors. Artifacts in MR imaging can result from anything that disrupts the T2* imaging signal, and may be caused by the MR scanner hardware or patient interaction.[22]

Motion-related artifacts can be random or episodic (essential tremor, breathing, cardiac related) and are usually minor in amplitude. As such, most fMR imaging postprocessing software packages are robust enough to remove noise and adequately coregister BOLD and structural MR imaging series. Stimulus-related motion (eg, facial movement during word generation or sentence rhyming) can be difficult to remove. With modern statistical analysis, these motion-related signal artifacts may be removed as long as they vary enough from signal generated by the stimulus presentation. It is noteworthy that significant motion artifact can limit the BOLD series' diagnostic value and can be difficult to remove with standard motion correction. This artifact can affect stimulus-related BOLD signal and structural correlation, and be mistaken for the stimulus-generated signal, adversely affecting the study.[1] A strategy to overcome this limitation is to use the contralateral hemisphere as a reference control to simplify suppositions about displaced anatomy and affected BOLD signal magnitudes.[23] In such cases, repeat acquisition is recommended.

The BOLD fMR imaging signal can be attenuated by noise. Multi-echo echo-planar (EP) imaging, whereby the fMR imaging signal is collected at multiple echo times, is a method to improve sensitivity to BOLD responses.[24] This allows for better noise reduction capability and offers advantages in imaging brain regions susceptible to distortion and signal dropout.[24] It is important to routinely inspect T2*-weighted images in an attempt to correct any and all artifacts found during the fMR imaging scans. As BOLD fMR imaging is an EP imaging–based technique, susceptibility artifact can result in BOLD signal loss, for example in blood products (hemosiderin), air-tissue interface, and metal (eg, dental hardware, surgical hardware near cortical regions).[1]

Neurovascular uncoupling (NVU), which refers to disruption of coupling between neuronal activity and neurovascular response in areas within or surrounding the tumor, is a major pitfall to consider, as it can lead to false-negative neuronal activity. The BOLD effect is proportional to the net change in volume from oxygenated to deoxygenated blood in the tissue; this is true as long as the natural HRF between the neurovascular system and the brain is preserved. In certain conditions—for example, hypervascular neoplasms—the normal HRF is disrupted, predisposing to NVU. As such, lesions in the eloquent cortex with marked increased vascularity should be scrutinized closely in cases demonstrating limited to no significant neuronal activation.[1]

BLOOD-OXYGEN-LEVEL–DEPENDENT FUNCTIONAL MR IMAGING APPLICATIONS

BOLD fMR imaging can reliably map eloquent cortex presurgically and is sufficiently accurate for neurosurgical planning. HRF captured on BOLD fMR imaging allows for noninvasive in vivo assessment of eloquent cortical activation.[25] BOLD fMR imaging is useful for identification of the primary sensorimotor cortex, especially in cases where gyral anatomy is distorted by neoplasm or other CNS disorder (see **Fig. 1**). In patients with brain tumors undergoing neurosurgical intervention, fMR imaging can decrease postoperative morbidity by identifying eloquent cortex prospectively to guide surgical intervention. BOLD fMR imaging can be performed to evaluate the sensorimotor regions with paradigms that are both volitional and passive.[26] Normal brain anatomic variance (see **Fig. 1**) is another reason patients undergo fMR imaging, because the conventional anatomic landmarks associated with functional brain regions cannot be identified on structural imaging.[26,27]

Neuroplasticity refers to the reorganization of neural networks that can be seen in the setting of slow-growing neoplasms and is another key factor to be considered in functional recovery of patients with brain tumors. fMR imaging can help identify reorganization in cerebral networks prospectively, guiding appropriate surgical intervention and minimizing postoperative morbidity.[28] In patients with CNS neoplasms and history of stroke or comorbidities (eg, hypertension, coronary artery disease, diabetes) placing them at risk for stroke, fMR imaging can help depict reorganization of functional networks. Studies have shown that performing simple motor tasks with the affected limb following a stroke is associated with higher brain activation in many cortical areas when compared with healthy volunteers, including regions of the dorsal motor cortex, the ventral motor cortex, and the SMA.[28] Longitudinal fMR imaging studies have revealed that neural activity is often enhanced in motion-related areas in both hemispheres before returning to normal levels similar to those in healthy controls during the first 12 months after stroke.[3]

Numerous other considerations are important when performing BOLD fMR imaging in clinical practice. For example, patients with brain tumors benefit from shorter-length tasks because they find greater difficulty keeping their head still in comparison with healthy subjects. Numerous studies have shown that patients benefit from signal averaging via block design, meaning that brain regions associated with a specific task can be activated even if it is not essential to the task being performed.[29] For example, since the primary visual cortex shows robust activation on language fMR imaging paradigms, the authors reduce the overall scan time in patients in whom the visual cortex is uninvolved by acquiring information of the primary visual cortex on language paradigms and excluding visual paradigms from the fMR imaging examinations. The authors perform fMR imaging examinations with dedicated visual paradigms in cases where the patient is symptomatic (visual deficits), or when the primary visual cortical region is infiltrated by neoplasm or distorted by mass effect. Similarly, in instances when eloquent cortex is distant from pathology and functional deficits are not clinically detected, fMR imaging examinations are curtailed to reduce scan time for patient comfort. This strategy is also helpful in instances where the patient is projected to undergo a longer than usual MR imaging evaluation (eg, MR imaging spectroscopy).

BOLD fMR imaging in the postoperative setting is especially helpful if a patient is expected to undergo staged and/or multistep surgical resection. For example, after a tumor is removed, regions of brain compressed by mass effect may demonstrate regained functionality because this tissue can become active, showing the BOLD effect on postoperative fMR imaging.

TASK-BASED VERSUS RESTING-STATE BLOOD-OXYGEN-LEVEL–DEPENDENT FUNCTIONAL MR IMAGING

To elicit neuronal activation for generation of BOLD signal, patients are trained before entering the MR imaging scanner and instructed to follow tasks delivered in functional paradigms given as visual cues. For motor cortex activation (see **Fig. 2**), foot movement, finger tapping, and lip pucker (or tongue movement) are most commonly used. For language network assessment (**Fig. 6**), silent word generation, sentence completion, and rhyming are the 3 most commonly used paradigms. To limit scan variability, the American Society of Functional Neuroradiology has provided a list of paradigms with recommended scanner parameters (https://www.asfnr.org/paradigms/).

Task-fMR imaging depends on the patient's ability to perform specific tasks that elicit BOLD signal alternation on MR imaging. The BOLD series is overlaid on the structural imaging (usually high-resolution T1 and/or T2-weighted sequence) to locate eloquent regions such as the primary language and motor and visual cortices.[1–3] There are several Food and Drug Administration–approved commercial software packages available in clinical practice that have made evaluation of task-based fMR imaging less time consuming by automating most of the postprocessing (eg, motion correction, image registration).

Though reliable in most clinical settings, task-based fMR imaging presents certain limitations and disadvantages. For example, task-based fMR imaging cannot be performed in patients suffering from severe neurologic deficits (eg, dementia, complete paresis).[30] Depending on language limitations and/or educational barriers, several different tasks may be required to assess different motor and language functions. Many trials may be required to achieve the desired activation maps, resulting in lengthy scanning sessions.[30] Task-fMR imaging also has limited utility in the pediatric preadolescent setting (especially infants and toddlers) because of the required cooperation by patients, as these subjects cannot follow commands on task-paradigms that are usually delivered through visual cues.

rs-fMR imaging is another BOLD fMR imaging technique with potential for overcoming task-based limitations. rs-fMR imaging measures the BOLD effect over a period of time while the patient is in the MR scanner. Agarwal and colleagues[31] had originally measured the resting state of the human brain motor cortex with fMR imaging and discovered that even during rest, different brain regions are able to communicate without an actively performed task. Because there are no prescan training requirements of the subject for rs-fMR imaging scanning, patients can be instructed to lie quietly with their eyes closed during the scanning process.[31] rs-fMR imaging is emerging as a useful alternative to task-fMR imaging, especially in cases where task-fMR imaging cannot be performed. In the absence of task performance, rs-fMR imaging maps acquire BOLD signal corresponding to low-frequency neuronal signal fluctuations during rest, thus allowing for detection of multiple functional networks.[31] By using the changes in the BOLD signal, a 4-dimensional time series of the brain can be constructed to reflect changing neuronal activity.[6] As the data are processed through a series of steps including head motion correction, spatial smoothing, and

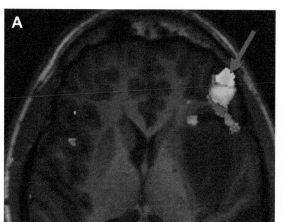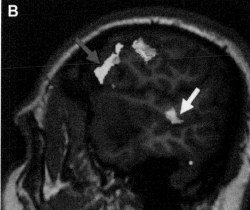

Fig. 6. A 42-year-old man with left insular glioma presented for presurgical language network mapping. fMR imaging depicts left cerebral dominance of the language network with robust activation in (*A*) Broca region (*red arrow*) and (*B*) Wernicke region (*yellow arrow*).

noise and bandpass filtering, the data can be evaluated.[6] Multiple subject comparison requires normalization of the data across all subjects followed by a method of targeting the connection between the regions.

The most popular analysis methods for targeting connections include seed-based analysis (SBA) and independent component analysis (ICA). SBA is a hypothesis-driven method that uses an extracted BOLD time course from the region of interest (ROI) to determine the connectivity of a seed relative to the rest of the brain.[32] ICA is a mathematical technique used to define a region of functional connectivity. ICA is a data-driven technique used to decompose the data set into independent components with strong temporal coherence (intraconnected maps), each of which associates with the time course of the overall signal.[4,32] Although the application of fMR imaging in neuro-oncology has become standard in localizing brain regions before surgery, there has been difficulty in transitioning from task-based localization to the resting state.

A key limitation in rs-fMR imaging has been the lack of standardization across many recent studies. Although new fMR imaging technologies are being developed, there is a lack of standardization of physiologic parameters, pharmacologic interventions, and characterization of disease-related vascular changes, with limited concrete data on how these changes affect the BOLD signal.[33] Current methods to analyze data also have limitations. SBA is based on predetermined ROIs, which can be arbitrary or task-fMR imaging derived.[24] Because some patients may have brain-distorting mass lesions, the collective database of ROIs may become difficult to use.[6,24] Although the uses of task versus rs-fMR imaging techniques differ in reliability to functional mapping, certain approaches see similar reliability with respect to mapping the sensorimotor network of healthy subjects. rs-fMR imaging has shown great promise as a diagnostic tool, and with enough comparative studies showing lack of discrepancy between both task and rs-fMR imaging, it has potential to become the noninvasive standard of care for surgical planning and prognosis.[30–33]

COMBINATION FUNCTIONAL BRAIN IMAGING

For presurgical planning, many techniques can be implemented complementarily to fMR imaging. Techniques used in place of or in addition to fMR imaging are magnetoencephalography (MEG), electroencephalography (EEG), PET, and diffusion tractography (DTI).[1] Different techniques can vary in spatial or temporal resolution, invasiveness, and how they localize or lateralize function.

MEG has been shown to predict the location of the gyrus of interest more accurately and specifically in comparison with fMR imaging.[34] Because fMR imaging activates the entire network (both primary and secondary areas) for motor tasks, there is difficulty interpreting where the primary, secondary, and sensory gyri are localized because they are acting simultaneously. This is not an issue with MEG. Spatial resolution between the 2 methods vary such that fMR imaging can be as low as 1 mm, whereas MEG achieves 5 mm.[34–36] Both techniques assist in more precise preoperative surgical planning compared with traditional MR markers, however, because MEG scanners are not as readily available as conventional MR imaging scanners, the latter being more commonly used.[1]

EEG is a method similar to MEG in that it directly measures electrical activity of the brain through small metal electrodes.[34] Even though intraoperative EEG is traditionally more invasive than fMR imaging, integrating the 2 techniques into the neurosurgical navigation system is beneficial in certain cases.

DTI is an MR technique that measures water diffusivity along white matter tracts using eigenvectors.[2,3] In particular, DTI is able to map and characterize diffusion as a function of spatial localization.[2,3] The combination of DTI with other imaging methods can improve its specificity for complex diseases. Combining DTI with gray matter fMR imaging localization paints a more complete picture of the functional anatomy in the area surrounding a tumor, with feedback such as tissue infiltration, distortion, and/or destruction.[1–3]

PET imaging can provide functional information by using a radioactive imaging agent conjugated with another compound (eg, glucose, antibodies, small molecules) depending on the disease of interest.[20,37] Fluorodeoxyglucose (FDG), a glucose analog, is the most commonly used PET radiotracer that provides metabolic information associated with tumor. FDG PET's role is somewhat limited in the setting of CNS neoplasms because there is increased background brain parenchymal FDG uptake resulting from physiologic neuronal activity, which limits spatial discrimination between tumor and adjacent normal brain tissue.[38] PET-MR imaging is a hybrid technology allowing for simultaneous acquisition of both PET and MR.[39] The benefit of the PET-MR imaging is that it can provide improved spatial resolution of detected CNS abnormalities with less (about 50%) PET radiotracer-associated radiation exposure.[39] In CNS disorders, PET-MR imaging scans are most commonly used for evaluation of neoplasms, epilepsy, and neurodegenerative disorders.

SUMMARY

Functional neuroimaging is integral to current clinical practice in various disciplines including neuro-oncology, neurodegenerative disorders, and epilepsy. BOLD fMR imaging has been shown to help in presurgical planning, minimizing the risk of postsurgical morbidity while reducing operative time and decreasing craniotomy size.[3,6] Task-based BOLD fMR imaging is the most commonly used technique for noninvasive assessment of eloquent cortex[2,3,6] and can reliably elucidate cortical regions involved in sensorimotor, language, and visual functions. Though reliable, it is important to be aware of pitfalls of this technique, such as neurovascular uncoupling and susceptibility artifact, so as to provide the most accurate functional assessment.

ACKNOWLEDGMENTS

Funding support: Dr A.A. Chaudhry received funding support from NIH 5K12CA001727-23 and City of Hope Young Investigator Award. The authors would like to acknowledge Seth Hilliard for his assistance with the literature search on this article.

REFERENCES

1. Gabriel M, Brennan NP, Peck KK, et al. Blood oxygen level dependent functional magnetic resonance imaging for presurgical planning. Neuroimaging Clin N Am 2014;24(4):557–71.
2. Ulmer JL, Klein AP, Mueller WM, et al. Preoperative diffusion tensor imaging: improving neurosurgical outcomes in brain tumor patients. Neuroimaging Clin N Am 2014;24(4):599–617.
3. Filippi M, Agosta F. Diffusion tensor imaging and functional MRI. Handb Clin Neurol 2016;136:1065–87.
4. Yeh CJ, Tseng YS, Lin YR, et al. Resting-state functional magnetic resonance imaging: the impact of regression analysis. J Neuroimaging 2015;25(1):117–23.
5. Buchbinder BR. Functional magnetic resonance imaging. Handb Clin Neurol 2016;135:61–92.
6. Lang S, Duncan N, Northoff G. Resting-state functional magnetic resonance imaging: review of neurosurgical applications. Neurosurgery 2014;74(5):453–64 [discussion: 464–5].
7. Dimou S, Battisti RA, Hermens DF, et al. A systematic review of functional magnetic resonance imaging

8. and diffusion tensor imaging modalities used in presurgical planning of brain tumour resection. Neurosurg Rev 2013;36(2):205–14 [discussion: 214].
8. Buxton RB. The physics of functional magnetic resonance imaging (fMRI). Rep Prog Phys 2013;76(9):096601.
9. Mangraviti A, Casali C, Cordella R, et al. Practical assessment of preoperative functional mapping techniques: navigated transcranial magnetic stimulation and functional magnetic resonance imaging. Neurol Sci 2013;34(9):1551–7.
10. Barras CD, Asadi H, Baldeweg T, et al. Functional magnetic resonance imaging in clinical practice: state of the art and science. Aust Fam Physician 2016;45(11):798–803.
11. Borich MR, Brodie SM, Gray WA, et al. Understanding the role of the primary somatosensory cortex: opportunities for rehabilitation. Neuropsychologia 2015;79(Pt B):246–55.
12. Silva MA, See AP, Essayed WI, et al. Challenges and techniques for presurgical brain mapping with functional MRI. Neuroimage Clin 2018;17:794–803.
13. Leisman G, Moustafa AA, Shafir T. Thinking, walking, talking: integratory motor and cognitive brain function. Front Public Health 2016;4:94.
14. Reid LB, Boyd RN, Cunnington R, et al. Interpreting intervention induced neuroplasticity with fMRI: the case for multimodal imaging strategies. Neural Plast 2016;2016:2643491.
15. Hassa T, de Jel E, Tuescher O, et al. Functional networks of motor inhibition in conversion disorder patients and feigning subjects. Neuroimage Clin 2016;11:719–27.
16. Potgieser AR, de Jong BM, Wagemakers M, et al. Insights from the supplementary motor area syndrome in balancing movement initiation and inhibition. Front Hum Neurosci 2014;8:960.
17. Vergani F, Lacerda L, Martino J, et al. White matter connections of the supplementary motor area in humans. J Neurol Neurosurg Psychiatry 2014;85(12):1377–85.
18. Yu ZB, Lv YB, Song LH, et al. Functional connectivity differences in the insular sub-regions in migraine without aura: a resting-state functional magnetic resonance imaging study. Front Behav Neurosci 2017;11:124.
19. Abalkhail TM, MacDonald DB, Al Thubaiti I, et al. Intraoperative direct cortical stimulation motor evoked potentials: stimulus parameter recommendations based on rheobase and chronaxie. Clin Neurophysiol 2017;128(11):2300–8.
20. Benjamin CFA, Dhingra I, Li AX, et al. Presurgical language fMRI: technical practices in epilepsy surgical planning. Hum Brain Mapp 2018;39(10):4032–42.
21. Szaflarski JP, Gloss D, Binder JR, et al. Practice guideline summary: use of fMRI in the presurgical

evaluation of patients with epilepsy: report of the guideline development, dissemination, and implementation Subcommittee of the American Academy of Neurology. Neurology 2017;88(4):395–402.

22. Krupa K, Bekiesinska-Figatowska M. Artifacts in magnetic resonance imaging. Pol J Radiol 2015; 80:93–106.

23. Middlebrooks EH, Frost CJ, Tuna IS, et al. Reduction of motion artifacts and noise using independent component analysis in task-based functional MRI for preoperative planning in patients with brain tumor. AJNR Am J Neuroradiol 2017;38(2):336–42.

24. Caballero-Gaudes C, Reynolds RC. Methods for cleaning the BOLD fMRI signal. Neuroimage 2017; 154:128–49.

25. Dewiputri WI, Auer T. Functional magnetic resonance imaging (FMRI) neurofeedback: implementations and applications. Malays J Med Sci 2013; 20(5):5–15.

26. Choudhri AF, Patel RM, Siddiqui A, et al. Cortical activation through passive-motion functional MRI. AJNR Am J Neuroradiol 2015;36(9):1675–81.

27. Durning SJ, Costanzo M, Artino AR Jr, et al. Using functional magnetic resonance imaging to improve how we understand, teach, and assess clinical reasoning. J Contin Educ Health Prof 2014;34(1): 76–82.

28. Li W, Wang M, Li Y, et al. A novel brain network construction method for exploring age-related functional reorganization. Comput Intell Neurosci 2016;2016: 2429691.

29. Abd-El-Barr MM, Saleh E, Huang RY, et al. Effect of disease and recovery on functional anatomy in brain tumor patients: insights from functional MRI and diffusion tensor imaging. Imaging Med 2013;5(4): 333–46.

30. Palacios EM, Sala-Llonch R, Junque C, et al. Resting-state functional magnetic resonance imaging activity and connectivity and cognitive outcome in traumatic brain injury. JAMA Neurol 2013;70(7): 845–51.

31. Agarwal S, Lu H, Pillai JJ. Value of frequency domain resting-state functional magnetic resonance imaging metrics amplitude of low-frequency fluctuation and fractional amplitude of low-frequency fluctuation in the assessment of brain tumor-induced neurovascular uncoupling. Brain Connect 2017;7(6):382–9.

32. Wu L, Caprihan A, Bustillo J, et al. An approach to directly link ICA and seed-based functional connectivity: application to schizophrenia. Neuroimage 2018;179:448–70.

33. Chen JE, Glover GH. Functional magnetic resonance imaging methods. Neuropsychol Rev 2015; 25(3):289–313.

34. Proudfoot M, Woolrich MW, Nobre AC, et al. Magnetoencephalography. Pract Neurol 2014;14(5): 336–43.

35. Schmid E, Thomschewski A, Taylor A, et al, E-PILEPSY consortium. Diagnostic accuracy of functional magnetic resonance imaging, Wada test, magnetoencephalography, and functional transcranial Doppler sonography for memory and language outcome after epilepsy surgery: a systematic review. Epilepsia 2018. https://doi.org/10.1111/epi.14588.

36. Sollmann N, Ille S, Boeckh-Behrens T, et al. Mapping of cortical language function by functional magnetic resonance imaging and repetitive navigated transcranial magnetic stimulation in 40 healthy subjects. Acta Neurochir (Wien) 2016;158(7):1303–16.

37. Bruinsma TJ, Sarma VV, Oh Y, et al. The relationship between dopamine neurotransmitter dynamics and the blood-oxygen-level-dependent (BOLD) Signal: a review of pharmacological functional magnetic resonance imaging. Front Neurosci 2018;12:238.

38. Smucny J, Wylie KP, Tregellas JR. Functional magnetic resonance imaging of intrinsic brain networks for translational drug discovery. Trends Pharmacol Sci 2014;35(8):397–403.

39. Matthews R, Choi M. Clinical utility of positron emission tomography magnetic resonance imaging (PET-MRI) in gastrointestinal cancers. Diagnostics (Basel) 2016; 6(3). https://doi.org/10.3390/diagnostics6030035.

Imaging Glioblastoma Posttreatment

Progression, Pseudoprogression, Pseudoresponse, Radiation Necrosis

Sara B. Strauss, MD, Alicia Meng, MD, Edward J. Ebani, MD,
Gloria C. Chiang, MD*

KEYWORDS

- Glioblastoma • Pseudoprogression • Pseudoresponse • Radiation necrosis

KEY POINTS

- Various assessment guidelines for tumor progression, primarily designed for the purpose of phase 2 clinical trials, have been used over the course of the past several decades, with changes over time reflecting evolution in the approach to treatment and technological advances in imaging.
- Radiation necrosis and pseudoprogression are often thought of as 2 opposite extremes on the spectrum of radiation-induced injury, and imaging features may mimic disease progression.
- Pseudoresponse occurs in the setting of antiangiogenic therapy, and imaging findings include decreased contrast enhancement, edema, and permeability as early as 1 day after initiation of therapy.
- A multimodality approach to treatment response coupled with an understanding of the strengths and limitations of various imaging techniques is essential to accurate assessment of treatment response.

INTRODUCTION

Eighty percent of all malignant primary brain tumors diagnosed in the United States are gliomas.[1] The current treatment paradigm for high-grade gliomas (grades III and IV) includes maximal surgical resection followed by concurrent adjuvant radiation and chemotherapy. The relatively recent addition of adjuvant chemotherapy with an oral alkylating agent, temozolomide, is based on pivotal data published in 2005 by Stupp and colleagues,[2] which demonstrated a clinically meaningful and statistically significant overall survival benefit with minimal additional toxicity.

For patients with primary treatment failure or recurrence, the Food and Drug Administration approved the use of bevacizumab, an anti–vascular endothelial growth factor (VEGF) monoclonal antibody, in 2009.[3] In addition, there are many experimental therapies currently under active investigation for patients with recurrent glioblastoma. These include immunomodulatory approaches, such as immune checkpoint inhibitors, tumor vaccines, chimeric antigen receptor (CAR)-modified T-cell therapy, and oncolytic virotherapy. Recently developed immune checkpoint inhibitors such as anti-CTLA-4 (ipilimumab) and anti-PD-1 (pembrolizumab and nivolumab) antibodies have demonstrated clinical efficacy in several solid tumors, with clinical trials for glioblastoma ongoing. Examples of viruses currently under investigation in patients with recurrent glioblastoma include an

Disclosure Statement: The authors have no conflicts of interest to disclose.
Department of Radiology, Weill Cornell Medical Center, 525 East 68th Street, Box 141, New York, NY 10065, USA
* Corresponding author.
E-mail address: gcc9004@med.cornell.edu

radiologic.theclinics.com

adenovirus expressing interleukin (IL)-12, a herpes simplex virus–1 replicating strain expressing IL-12, vaccine strains of the measles virus, an attenuated poliovirus vaccine, and a replicating retrovirus. Finally, alternating electric field therapy in which a portable device is attached to the scalp and delivers continuous low-intensity alternating electric fields has demonstrated prolonged progression-free and overall survival when used in combination with standard therapy. The device was approved in 2015 for the treatment of newly diagnosed glioblastoma and is expected to change the standard of care.[4]

Tumor recurrence occurs in patients within a median of 6.7 months,[5] with mean overall survival time of 14 to 16 months for glioblastomas.[2,6] Radiographic monitoring of response is key, with a recent publication proposing a standardized reporting template for posttreatment glioma, including tumor genetics (isocitrate dehydrogenase [IDH], O^6-methylguanine-DNA methyltransferase [MGMT] promoter) and treatment history.[7] The purpose of this review was to detail the imaging appearance of 4 key diagnoses in posttreatment glioma surveillance: true progression, pseudoprogression, pseudoresponse, and radiation necrosis.

CONVENTIONAL IMAGING: EVOLUTION OF ASSESSMENT CRITERIA
Progress

Various assessment guidelines for tumor progression, primarily designed for the purpose of phase 2 clinical trials, have been used over the course of the past several decades. Changes over time reflect evolution in the approach to treatment and technological advances in imaging.

The Levin criteria was a numerical grading system introduced in 1977, and imaging features important to diagnosis included size of tumor, central lucency, degree of contrast enhancement, surrounding edema, and ventricle size.[8] In 1990, the Macdonald criteria were published, relying heavily on maximal cross-sectional tumor measurements; these became the most widely used assessment guidelines for the ensuing 20 years.[9,10] The 2-dimensional approach to lesion measurement of the Macdonald criteria was replaced with the application of unidimensional measurement in the Response Evaluation Criteria in Solid Tumors (RECIST) guidelines to gliomas, defining progression by at least a 20% increase in the sum of the diameters of all target lesions, with a maximum of 5 lesions targeted for measurement.[11]

In 2010, the RANO (Response Assessment in Neurooncology) guidelines were introduced, and

progression was defined based on imaging features as well as time from completion of chemoradiation (<12 weeks and >12 weeks); important factors in determining progression included enhancement outside of the radiation field, increase by 25% or greater in the sum of the products of perpendicular diameters between the first post-radiotherapy (RT) scan and the scan 12 weeks later, or clinical deterioration. The RANO guidelines additionally consider use of anti-angiogenics; increase in T2/fluid-attenuated inversion recovery (FLAIR) signal in nonenhancing lesions in such patients is indicative of disease progression.[12] With the increased use of immunotherapy, the RANO in immunotherapy guidelines were introduced, which defined imaging criteria less than 6 months and more than 6 months after start of immunotherapy,[13] given that there may be a latency period during which disease may actually worsen while the effective immune response evolves.[14] Importantly, increase or decrease in steroid dose within 2 weeks of MR imaging assessment make disease progression nonevaluable according to the iRANO criteria.[13] The modified RANO criteria were published in 2017 with increased focus on pseudoprogression, and with progressive disease determination based on at least 2 sequential studies, separated by 4 weeks, showing 25% or more increase in size; any new measurable lesion requires confirmation on a repeat study 4 weeks later, clear clinical deterioration, or lack of repeat evaluation due to deteriorating condition/death.[15] The RANO criteria and subsequent modifications highlight the quandary behind many posttreatment glioma cases: both true disease progression and pseudoprogression can present with increased tumor enhancement. In fact, new enhancement seen within the radiation field within the first 12 weeks after treatment can never be definitively diagnosed as progression versus pseudoprogression based on the RANO guidelines.

The following sections cover both conventional and advanced imaging approaches to differentiating between these various entities.

DEFINITION OF PSEUDOPROGRESSION

Pseudoprogression is defined as radiographic evidence of disease progression, typically within 3 to 6 months posttreatment, followed by spontaneous resolution or improvement without additional treatment.[16,17] Pseudoprogression may be accompanied by symptoms in 21% to 34% of patients with high-grade gliomas, but may be asymptomatic in patients with low-grade gliomas, particularly in the adult population.[18] The pathophysiology of pseudoprogression is distinct from radiation necrosis, and likely relates to endothelial cell injury resulting in tissue inflammation and upregulation of VEGF leading to increased vessel permeability and edema, an effect potentiated by chemotherapy administration.[16] In addition to high-grade gliomas, low-grade (World Health Organization [WHO] II) gliomas and WHO III (IDH mutant) gliomas also can demonstrate pseudoprogression.[19–21] Studies have shown that ultimately, patients with pseudoprogression have better outcomes,[20,22] presumably because pseudoprogression reflects an augmented response to treatment.

Early recognition of the concept of pseudoprogression in the setting of radiotherapy led to the suggestion that patients with radiological evidence of progressive disease within the first 3 months of treatment be excluded from phase 2 trials.[23] It was subsequently learned that concurrent treatment with RT and chemotherapy potentiated the effects of radiation necrosis,[24] leading to earlier manifestation of pseudoprogression after treatment initiation. Misinterpretation of pseudoprogression is problematic in terms of patient assignment to clinical trials, interpretation of trial results, guidance of decisions regarding reoperation, and in contributing to patient anxiety.[25] Prospective identification of pseudoprogression can be radiologically and even histologically challenging,[26] and inconsistency in the definition of pseudoprogression confounds comparison between studies. **Figs. 1** and **2** illustrate examples of biopsy-proven progression and pseudoprogression, respectively.

FACTORS ASSOCIATED WITH PSEUDOPROGRESSION

Factors associated with pseudoprogression include cancer genotype and radiation dose. MGMT methylation is associated with increased probability of pseudoprogression and better outcomes.[27–29] For instance, in a group of 157 patients with glioblastoma multiforme, IDH1 mutation, and MGMT methylation predicted a high probability of pseudoprogression, as well as improved overall survival.[30] The incidence of pseudoprogression in patients with MGMT methylated tumor genetics was shown to be 91% compared with 41% in patients with the unmethylated promotor.[31] IDH1 mutation was shown to have high specificity in the detection of pseudoprogression in a study of 32 patients with GBM treated with temozolomide and radiotherapy.[32] Dose of radiotherapy also impacts likelihood of pseudoprogression[2,16] and among patients with lower-grade glioma, proton therapy results in higher prevalence

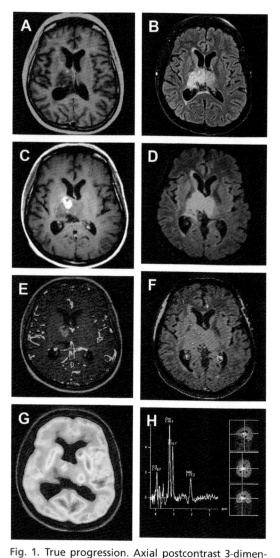

Fig. 1. True progression. Axial postcontrast 3-dimensional T1 SPACE (*A, C*) and T2 FLAIR images (*B, D*) demonstrating a bithalamic infiltrative anaplastic astrocytoma (*B*) with a small enhancing nodule in the right anterior thalamus (*A*). A month later, the enhancing nodule increased significantly in size (*C*), with increased T2 hyperintensity and local mass effect (*D*). DCE-MR perfusion was performed to help evaluate the degree of tumor angiogenesis. Region-of-interest interrogation of the enhancing nodule on the Vp map, superimposed on the postcontrast T1 (*E*), demonstrated markedly elevated plasma volume relative to contralateral thalamus and normal-appearing white matter. As evident on the Ktrans map, superimposed on the T2 FLAIR (*F*), there was also associated elevated permeability. An image from the integrated PET-MR study demonstrated elevated FDG uptake in the enhancing nodule (*G*). Single-voxel MRS (*H*) demonstrated an elevated choline-to-NAA ratio, also compatible with tumor metabolism. Subsequent surgical biopsy confirmed tumor progression.

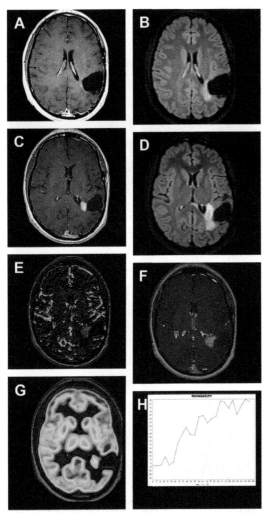

Fig. 2. Pseudoprogression. Axial postcontrast T1 (*A, C*) and T2 FLAIR images (*B, D*) demonstrate a small focus of enhancement along the medial margin of the resection cavity (*A*) and surrounding T2 hyperintensity extending to the ependymal margin of the left lateral ventricle (*B*). The patient had a pathologically proven oligodendroglioma and had undergone proton beam radiation therapy, completed 5 months prior, and several cycles of procarbazine/lomustine. On subsequent imaging, the enhancing nodule had grown (*C*) and there was increased surrounding T2 hyperintensity (*D*). DCE-MR perfusion was performed to help differentiate between tumor progression and radiation necrosis. Region-of-interest interrogation of the enhancing nodule on the Vp map, superimposed on the postcontrast T1 (*E*), demonstrated an elevated plasma volume, approximately double that of normal-appearing white matter. There was also associated elevated permeability (*F, H*). An image from the integrated PET-MR study (*G*) demonstrated that the enhancing nodule had FDG uptake that was greater than adjacent white matter, but less than normal cortex. Subsequent surgical biopsy confirmed radiation-related changes.

of pseudoprogression compared with photon therapy among patients with oligodendroglioma, but not astrocytoma, and pseudoprogression is associated with better progression-free survival.[22] Therefore, these factors have important implications for the interpretation of posttreatment imaging,[33,34] and the diagnostic accuracy of advanced imaging.[35] Interestingly, age and size of the treated lesion were shown to be unrelated to likelihood of pseudoprogresssion.[36] Prospective identification of pseudoprogression is a challenging exercise, and even use of both conventional and advanced imaging techniques may not consistently result in success.[37]

DIFFERENTIATING PSEUDOPROGRESSION FROM TRUE PROGRESSION

Immediate postsurgical imaging should take place within 48 hours postoperatively, in order to avoid postprocedural confounders such as enhancement associated with subacute ischemia.[38] Subsequent follow-up imaging typically takes place after completion of chemoradiation, usually over the course of 6 weeks.

On conventional imaging, enhancement pattern and signal intensity on T2-weighted images are important factors in diagnosing tumor recurrence. Several studies have identified specific enhancement patterns that can aid in elaborating degree of suspicion of true tumor progression. Mullins and colleagues[39] found that involvement of the corpus callosum was most predictive of progression, and that likelihood of tumor progression increased when callosal involvement was seen in combination with multiple enhancing lesions, crossing of the midline, and subependymal spread. Similarly, subependymal enhancement was shown to be predictive of true progression with 93.3% specificity in a retrospective study of 93 patients with GBM undergoing chemoradiation who developed new or increased enhancing mass lesions. However, no features on conventional imaging were found to have high negative predictive value for pseudoprogression.[40] Subependymal enhancement, specifically at a distance from the primary enhancing lesion (>1 cm), was shown to be more common in true progression than pseudoprogression.[41] Focal solid nodular enhancement and solid uniform enhancement with distinct margins was seen in 85% of patients with histopathologically proven tumor recurrence in a group of 51 patients who underwent reoperation after completing chemoradiation.[42]

Increased T2/FLAIR signal is another important qualitative criterion for tumor progression, but can also be seen in the setting of pseudoprogression, secondary to tissue injury or laminar necrosis. However, enhancement in the absence of edema on T2-weighted images is suggestive of pseudoprogression.[43] Signal change extending to cortex and mass effect are more suggestive of tumor progression than pseudoprogression.[44] Increased FLAIR volume and extension beyond the radiation field are also clues to true progression as compared with pseudoprogression.[45] In fact, a postmortem analysis demonstrated that T2-weighted images were most representative of tumor extent compared with postcontrast T1-weighted images when correlated with histopathologic specimens.[46]

Despite heavy reliance on conventional imaging for progression guidelines and attention to subtleties in postcontrast T1 and FLAIR appearance, the sensitivity and specificity of anatomic MR imaging for detection of progression is low. In a recent meta-analysis of 5 studies, including 166 patients, the pooled sensitivity and specificity for anatomic MR imaging was 68% (95% confidence interval [CI] 51–81) and 77% (45–93), respectively, with better performance calculated for advanced imaging techniques (diffusion-weighted imaging [DWI], perfusion-weighted imaging [PWI], and magnetic resonance spectroscopy [MRS]).[37] Ultimately, multimodal assessment might be most productive in differentiating progression from pseudoprogression.[47–51]

MAGNETIC RESONANCE PERFUSION
Perfusion-Weighted Imaging

Three methods are used for PWI, 2 of which rely on the injection of an extrinsic contrast medium (dynamic susceptibility contrast [DSC] and dynamic contrast enhancement [DCE]), and 1 that uses blood as an intrinsic contrast medium (arterial spin labeling [ASL]). In a recent survey conducted by the American Society of Neuroradiology, 151 of 195 institutions endorsed offering perfusion MR imaging and 87% included perfusion as part of the standard brain tumor protocol, with percentage increase to 96% in the evaluation of pseudoprogression[52]; this compared with 48% of a total of 220 health centers across 31 European countries according to a European Society of Neuroradiology survey.[53] DSC was more commonly used than DCE and ASL; and only half of the institutions endorsed quantitative analysis. DSC perfusion, evaluated in 18 studies including 708 patients, had a sensitivity of 87% (82–91) with a specificity of 86% (77–91). DCE-perfusion evaluated in 5 studies including 207 patients had a sensitivity of 92% (73–98) and specificity of 85% (76–92).[52]

Dynamic Susceptibility Contrast

DSC is the most widely used technique for PWI[37]; in a study comparing all 3 perfusion methods, DSC was found to have the best diagnostic performance.[54] DSC relies on T2 and T2* signal changes related to the passage of a paramagnetic contrast agent, and aims at characterizing the hemodynamic properties of the central nervous system microvasculature. A loss of signal versus time curve for every voxel is generated, from which several functional maps are derived. Cerebral blood volume (CBV) is the most commonly used parameter, defined as milliliters of blood per 100 g of brain tissue, and is usually discussed relative to the contralesional brain tissue; this parameter is a surrogate marker for capillary density/neoangiogenesis. Cerebral blood flow (CBF) is the amount of blood in a given volume of tissue per time (mL of blood/100 g brain tissue/min), and is interpreted as the microvascular blood flow in a given region of interest. Mean transit time (MTT) is calculated by dividing CBV by CBF (MTT = CBV/CBF), and is defined as the amount of time it takes for the injected contrast to travel through a defined region or volume of interest. Finally, time to peak is defined as the amount of time it takes for contrast to achieve peak concentration.[55]

Advantages of DSC include its relatively quick and facile execution; limitations include user-dependent calculation of absolute parameter measures and sensitivity to susceptibility-related artifact, particularly at the skull base or in the presence of postoperative hemosiderin deposition. Regional CBV (rCBV) measurements may differ in diagnostic accuracy based on the use of contrast preloading and baseline subtraction techniques.[56] Choice of software package has been shown to bear clinically significant differences in CBV.[57]

In high-grade gliomas, tumor growth leads to neovascularity, increased microvascular density, and slower flow in collateral vasculature, which translates into elevated CBV.[58,59] Multiple studies examining DSC-MR in the setting of posttreatment glioma demonstrate elevated rCBV in the setting of tumor progression.[33,50,54,60–66] Although a recent survey indicated that approximately 50% of surveyed institutions do not process quantitative parameter maps, published studies show that inspection of color maps in the absence of parameter computation does not reliably differentiate progression from psuedoprogression.[67] The challenge in a quantitative approach to DSC-MR is the lack of universal threshold, limiting reproducibility. This is underscored by the wide range of thresholds values for rCBV reported in the literature. For instance, Hu and colleagues[63] demonstrated that an rCBV cutoff value of 0.71 predicted true progression from pseudoprogression with 95.9% accuracy; however, the reported range of rCBV thresholds in the literature range from 0.9 to 2.15 for mean rCBV and 1.49 to 3.10 for maximum rCBV.[68,69] Interestingly, in a meta-analysis examining the utility of DSC perfusion in differentiating progression from pseudoprogression, Wang and colleagues[70] found that differences in threshold values had only a mild effect on individual study accuracy. Other approaches to parameter analysis include rCBV histogram skewness and kurtosis, tumor fractional volume,[68,71,72] parametric response mapping,[73,74] and evaluation of trends over time rather than static computations.[71,75]

Dynamic Contrast Enhancement

DCE is a T1-weighted sequence that usually uses spoiled gradient echo technique, requiring longer acquisition time compared with DSC. Longer acquisition times, ranging from 6 to 10 minutes,[76] are required to characterize the permeability of the blood brain barrier and its relationship to the extracellular extravascular space.[55] Concentration time curves are generated, from which several parameters can be calculated, including Ktrans, the rate of transfer between plasma and extravascular tissue; Kep, the rate of transfer between extravascular tissue and plasma; Ve, the extracellular volume; and Vp, the plasma volume.[77,78] Advantages of DCE include the increased information gained regarding microvascular permeability and blood brain barrier, as well as the technique's decreased sensitivity to susceptibility-related artifact. Disadvantages include the longer scan time, decreased temporal resolution, and differences of opinion regarding ideal pharmacokinetic modeling, which limit comparisons across sites. Compared with DSC, DCE has more limited temporal resolution but improved spatial resolution, and is therefore preferable for lesions with mixed pathology.[16]

The diagnostic accuracy for DCE was shown to be similar to DSC[69] in a meta-analysis performed by van Djiken and colleagues.[37] The expectation, confirmed by several retrospective[79] and prospective[80,81] studies, is that Ktrans and Vp are higher in the setting of true progression compared with pseudoprogression[79,81] and radiation necrosis.[68] Semiquantitative methods using area under the curve (AUC) also have been applied successfully in the evaluation of progression versus pseudoprogression.[82,83] In a retrospective study of 37 patients with GBM and new/increasing enhancement after treatment, Thomas and colleagues[79] determined that Vp (mean) cutoff less than 3.7 yielded 85% sensitivity and 79% specificity for pseudoprogression and Ktrans (mean) of greater than 3.6 had a 69% sensitivity and 79% specificity for disease progression; however, as with DSC, universal thresholds have not been established.[84]

Arterial Spin Labeling

ASL is a technique that uses a series of short radiofrequency pulses to label endogenous protons in arterial blood.[85] CBF is calculated based on the difference in signal between baseline images and the magnetically labeled images, and can be applied using a pseudocontinuous or pulsed technique.[86] Labeling time is approximately 2 to 4 seconds, followed by a 1.5-second to 2.0-second delay, after which signal is acquired by using fast spin echo or gradient echo technique.[77,78] The calculated parameter of interest is CBF, which has been shown to correlate well with rCBV generated using DCE technique, but, unlike DCE, leakage correction is not required.[86] Because of the intrinsically low signal to noise, ASL scan times are longer and therefore prone to motion artifact.[85,87] Moreover, complexity of ASL flow calculations make ASL a less popular perfusion technique.[87] Studies have demonstrated the utility of ASL as both an independent perfusion method[55] and as an adjunct to other perfusion methods such as DSC[88] in differentiating between progression and pseudoprogression; however, this method is less frequently used for reasons discussed previously.

DIFFUSION
Diffusion-Weighted Imaging

DWI is an MR imaging technique sensitive to the molecular motion of water through the addition of 2 identical diffusion gradients, one on each side of a 180° refocusing pulse[89]; increased cellularity in the setting of high-grade glioma confers high microscopic tissue organization, and is detected as reduced diffusion.[77] Apparent diffusion coefficient (ADC), a measure of water diffusivity, has therefore been used in the differentiation of tumor progression from pseudoprogression.[66,89–93]

DWI can be used as both a qualitative[90,93] and quantitative[91,94,95] imaging tool in differentiating progression from pseudoprogression. For instance, on the basis of visual inspection alone, Lee and colleagues[90] found that in a group of 22 patients with GBM treated with chemoradiation, the progression group showed a higher incidence of homogeneous or multifocal high signal intensity on diffusion-weighted images, whereas only peripheral hyperintensity or no high signal intensity was more frequently observed in the pseudoprogression group. Using a quantitative approach, multiple studies have shown that mean ADC values are lower in patients with true progression as compared with pseudoprogression[41,90,92,94]; relative similarity in thresholds has been demonstrated between studies.[91,92] ADC values are particularly useful in the setting of nonenhancing T2/FLAIR hyperintensity, as low ADC values have been shown to precede the appearance of enhancing, viable tumor by a median of 3 months in patients undergoing treatment for GBM.[96] In addition to qualitative diffusion features and mean ADC values, cumulative ADC histogram analysis has been shown to aid in the differentiation of true progression from pseudoprogression,[97–99] as have voxel-wise approaches using parametric response maps[95] and functional diffusion maps.[100]

Diffusion Tensor Imaging

Diffusion tensor imaging (DTI) is an MR imaging technique that is sensitive to not only the degree but the direction of water diffusion. The technique applies at least 6 noncollinear directions of diffusion sensitization; the number of diffusion sensitizing directions can vary from 6 to 256.[101] Multiple quantitative parameters can be calculated, including fractional anisotropy (FA), which is a summary measure reflecting the overall directional coherence of water.

Studies using DTI in posttreatment monitoring show mixed interpretation of diffusion parameters. Although one might expect higher FA in areas of true tumor progression compared with pseudoprogression, ostensibly due to increased cellularity and therefore tissue organization expected in high-grade glioma, the limited number of studies applying DTI in the setting of treatment response have shown inconsistent results, with studies showing no difference in FA,[102,103] higher FA,[70] and lower FA[104] values in true progression compared with pseudoprogression.

Magnetic Resonance Spectroscopy

MRS is a technique that identifies and quantifies particular metabolites in a lesion of interest. MRS can be performed using multi-voxel or single-voxel techniques, to generate a plot of signal to frequency, expressed in parts per million.[77,105,106] Clinically relevant metabolites include N-acetylaspartate (NAA), a marker of neuronal viability; total choline (tCho), a marker of cell membrane turnover/cellular proliferation; total creatine (tCr), an energy metabolite; lactate, a product of anaerobic glycolytic metabolism; and lipid (triglycerides), a marker of necrosis.[77,106] Given its stable concentration, creatine is used as the reference for report of the metabolites of interest,[107] and typically high-grade gliomas are characterized by elevation of tCho and decrease in NAA.[108–111]

Limitations of MRS are multiple. Single-voxel approaches are prone to partial volume effects,[112] and there is limited ability to detect smaller lesions. Because of low metabolite concentrations, multiple acquisitions are required necessitating long scan times and, finally, there is the technical onus of eliminating contamination from adjacent tissues, such as scalp and ventricle.[37] Nevertheless, in a pooled meta-analysis of 9 studies including 203 patients, van Dijken and colleagues[37] found that MRS had the highest accuracy in response evaluation compared with conventional MR imaging, DWI, and perfusion MR imaging, with sensitivity of spectroscopy reported at 91% (79–97) and specificity reported at 95% (65–99).

MRS is a useful tool in determining progression from pseudoprogression. In a longitudinal study, Sawlani and colleagues[113] used single-voxel MRS to show elevation of lipid peaks and decrease in tCho/NAA ratios in patients with pseudoprogression, whereas elevated Cho and elevated tCho/NAA ratio were seen in patients with true progression. In a prospective study of 24 patients with GBM, significant differences in MRS data were recorded for patients with progression and pseudoprogression, with ideal institutional recurrence thresholds established as tNAA $\leq$1.5 mM, tCho/tNAA $\geq$1.4 (sensitivity 100%, specificity 91.7%), tNAA/Cr $\leq$0.7[91]; the investigators subsequently validated these thresholds, and concluded that GBM relapse was characterized by the tCho/tNAA ratio $\geq$1.3 with sensitivity of 100% and specificity of 94.7% (P<.001).[92] However, some studies have shown that Cho and NAA are increased in both progression and pseudoprogression, particularly in the early post-radiation time point.[114] Recently, 2-hydroxyglutarate was noted to accumulate in tumors with the IDH mutation,[115] and this metabolite can be used to monitor response to treatment in IDH-mutated gliomas.[116]

PET with Fludeoxyglucose

The most widely used PET tracer is, 2-(18F) fluoro-2-deoxy-D-glucose (FDG), a glucose analog incorporated into glycolytic metabolism; FDG-PET is used to monitor treatment response in glioblastoma.[117–120] Standardized uptake values represent the ratio of radiotracer activity in tissue relative to the injected dose per kilogram of body weight. Limitations to FDG-PET include physiologic uptake in normal brain parenchyma, constraining evaluation of small lesions, in addition to the observation that some high-grade gliomas may have decreased FDG uptake, creating a confusing clinical picture.[121]

A meta-analysis of 18F-FDG-PET utility in detecting recurrence in glioma revealed pooled sensitivity of 0.77 (95% CI, 0.66–0.85) and specificity of 0.78 (95% CI, 0.54–0.91).[122] A wide range of standardized uptake value (SUV) cutoff values for detection of glioma recurrence are reported in the literature, ranging from 1.3 to 1.5 relative to normal white matter, 0.5 to 1.05 relative to normal gray matter, and 1.3 to 1.35 for a mirror-image location as a reference,[106] with equally varying degrees of sensitivity and specificity.[123]

The utility of radiolabeled amino acid PET tracers in the posttreatment setting has also been explored. 11C–MET PET/MR imaging has been shown to have greater sensitivity, specificity and AUC compared with FDG-PET[124] and compared with MR imaging alone.[122,125] However, 11C-MET has a short half-life and therefore requires an on-site cyclotron, limiting its practical use. O-(2–18FFluoroethyl)- L-tyrosine (18F-FET) has a longer half-life than 11C-MET, and has been similarly applied in treatment monitoring.[126–130] Disadvantages of 18F-FET include slower renal elimination, resulting in increased residual tracer in the blood pool and, therefore, nonspecific tracer uptake.[131]

PSEUDOPROGRESSION IN IMMUNOTHERAPY

In the setting of immunotherapy, increase in size of a treated lesion may reflect a localized inflammatory response induced by immunotherapy and apparent new, enhancing lesions may represent immune response in previously infiltrative, nonenhancing disease. Delayed response and/or a "flare phenomenon" may occur,[132,133] and a number of studies have been performed to explore the associated perfusion[134,135] and diffusion[135,136] changes. Application of MRS to treatment response in immunotherapy also has been explored,[137] and has been shown to aid in identification of pseudoprogression in the setting of new lesion enhancement. Because lipid is a substrate of natural killer T cells, a lipid peak on MRS may be seen in the setting of immunotherapy response.[77,138] The application of FDG-PET and ASL have been less well-explored, and remain important potential avenues for future research efforts.

PSEUDORESPONSE

Whereas pseudoprogression typically occurs in the setting of administration of radiation and an alkylating agent, pseudoresponse occurs in the setting of antiangiogenic therapy. Glioblastoma is a highly vascular tumor that depends on angiogenesis for growth, with upregulation of several proangiogenic factors, including VEGF, hepatocyte growth factor, fibroblast growth factor, platelet-derived growth factor, angiopoietins, and IL-8,[139] resulting in disorganized vasculature with abnormalities in endothelial wall, pericyte coverage, and basement membrane.[140] Bevacizumab is a humanized monoclonal antibody that targets and binds VEGF-A, a highly expressed proangiogenic factor in brain tumors.[139] By targeting VEGF, normalization of tumor vasculature occurs with decrease in vessel size and permeability. This alteration in vasculature is believed to improve delivery of chemotherapy and/or radiation therapy.[141]

Imaging findings after anti-VEGF therapy include decreased contrast enhancement, edema, and permeability as early as 1 day after initiation of therapy.[141] Radiologic response rates are high, ranging from 25% to 60%.[1,2] Despite remarkable imaging response following bevacizumab administration, there has been no proven substantial benefit in overall survival. Bevacizumab, however, has been shown to improve progression-free survival with decreased patient dependence on steroid treatment.[142] A large fraction of patients who initially demonstrate radiographic response eventually develop progressive disease in the form of worsening, nonenhancing T2 signal hyperintensity on T2 FLAIR sequences.[143] Although presence of increased T2 FLAIR signal in nonenhancing tumor during antiangiogenic therapy has been shown to be associated with a higher risk of death, the usage of T2 FLAIR monitoring has been controversial given variability in interpretation.[144]

Several imaging methods have been investigated to distinguish true response from pseudoresponse in the setting of antiangiogenic therapy. The utility of perfusion imaging has been explored with equivocal results. Stadlbauer and colleagues[145] pointed out the limitation of DSC perfusion, because both normal brain parenchyma and tumor exhibit decreased perfusion following bevacizumab administration. Other studies have demonstrated the utility of DSC perfusion in detecting decrease in permeability following antiangiogenic therapy, which correlated with overall survival or progression-free survival.[146,147]

Although ADC value is helpful in differentiating true progression from pseudoprogression, ADC

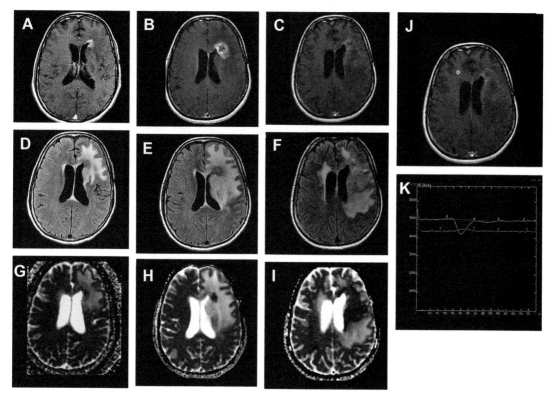

Fig. 3. Pseudoresponse. Axial postcontrast T1 (*A–C*), T2 FLAIR (*D–F*), and corresponding ADC maps showing the temporal progression of imaging findings of a glioblastoma that progressed and was subsequently treated with bevacizumab. The initial imaging demonstrated an area of enhancement along the left frontal horn (*A*), with surrounding T2 hyperintensity (*D*) likely representing a combination of infiltrative tumor, vasogenic edema, and/or treatment-related gliosis. A small focus of ADC hypointensity was also noted (*G*). A month later, both the enhancement (*B*) and T2 hyperintensity (*E*) progressed, with associated expansion of the area of ADC hypointensity (*H*), possibly reflecting hypercellular tumor. Bevacizumab therapy was started immediately after this scan. Two months later, the enhancement had decreased significantly (*C*), giving the appearance of a response to therapy. However, the area of heterogeneous T2 hyperintensity (*F*) and ADC hypointensity (*I*) further expanded. This was biopsy-proven to be viable tumor. Of note, DSC-MR perfusion was misleading by demonstrating no elevated CBV in the area of enhancement (*J, K*), likely given the antiangiogenic effect of the bevacizumab.

values may be of limited usefulness in evaluating pseudoresponse. A recent study of ADC values in patients on bevacizumab demonstrated normalization of ADC values following initiation of treatment that persisted even when progressive disease was reported.[148] However, preantiangiogenic treatment ADC values at a threshold of greater than 1.24 $\mu m^2/ms$ have been shown to predict improved overall survival in patients with recurrent glioblastoma.[149]

More recently, amino acid PET has shown promising ability to improve identification of viable tumor by detecting the tumor's demand for carbon. A case report cited the ability of radiolabeled amino acid 18F-FET PET to detect progressive tumors earlier in patients treated with bevacizumab.[150] Another study, investigating the use of radiolabeled 3,4-dihydroxy-6-[18F]-fluoro-L-phenylalanine (18F-FDOPA) PET found that

metabolic tumor volumes were predictive of treatment response and overall survival as early as 2 weeks following the initiation of bevacizumab.[151] **Fig. 3** illustrates the temporal progression of imaging findings of a glioblastoma treated with bevacizumab after tumor progression.

RADIATION NECROSIS

Radiation necrosis and pseudoprogression are often thought of as 2 opposite extremes along the spectrum of radiation-induced injury. The terms are often interchanged, and several studies examining progression versus "treatment-related change" refer to pseudoprogression and radiation necrosis as a single collective entity.[49,54,152–154] However, pseudoprogression and radiation necrosis are, in fact, distinct in timing, pathomechanism, histopathology, and prognosis. Pseudoprogression typically occurs within weeks to months after treatment, whereas radiation necrosis typically occurs 9 to 12 months after treatment and can occur up to several years later; new areas of contrast enhancement are typically bounded by the initial radiation field.[44] In pseudoprogression, vasodilation, perturbations in the blood brain barrier, and vasogenic edema lead to transient effects, whereas more severe injury in radiation necrosis related to oligodendrocyte injury, autoimmune mechanisms, and endothelial cell death leads to more irreversible fibrinoid necrosis, fibrosis, reactive gliosis, demyelination, and vascular hyalinization.[10,26,37] Perhaps the most important distinction between the two is that patients with pseudoprogression have a more favorable prognosis, whereas patients with radiation necrosis experience more profound neurologic decline and ultimately have a worse prognosis.[16] The frequency of radiation necrosis is reported anywhere from 5% to 25%, with risk proportionate to radiation dose,[16,155,156] with the 1p/19q codeletion shown to be a significant risk factor.[157] Treatment options for radiation necrosis include bevacizumab, anticoagulation, hyperbaric oxygen therapy, vitamin E, and laser interstitial thermal therapy.[10]

On conventional imaging, several imaging features are suggestive of radiation necrosis compared with progression. Radiation necrosis typically involves the periventricular white matter within or adjacent to the radiation field, due to its tenuous blood supply,[16] but can occur in a contralesional and multifocal distribution as well.[158] Internal enhancement patterns, described as "Swiss-cheese" or "soap-bubble," have been shown to be more typical of radiation necrosis,[158] as has the presence of diffuse, "meshlike enhancement" or peripheral enhancement with "feathery" margins.[42,159] On T2-weighted imaging, the central necrotic component will have high signal, whereas the solid component will have relatively lower signal.

Advanced imaging techniques available for differentiation between radiation necrosis and progression are similar to those applied in the early posttreatment period in evaluating for pseudoprogression[48,160] and include DWI,[161,162] PWI,[163] including DSC,[152,164] DCE,[154,165] and ASL,[166] MRS,[167–170] and PET.[171] In general, true progression will exhibit increased perfusion,[152,164,172] elevated rCBV,[173] lower ADC values on DWI,[41,104,161,172] higher Cho/Cr (choline/creatine) and Cho/NAA (choline/N-acetyl aspartate) ratios and lower NAA/Cr ratios,[77,160] and increased SUV uptake in true progression compared with radiation necrosis. The presence of a lipid peak is suggestive of radiation necrosis[77]; multivoxel MRS has been shown to be superior in diagnostic accuracy to single-voxel MRS, particularly in the setting of mixed pathology lesions.[174] There have been mixed results in terms of MRS and PET accuracy, and meta-analyses have shown moderate sensitivity and specificity for MRS,[175] 18F-FDG, and 11C-MET PET[122] in differentiating between progression and radiation necrosis. Kim and colleagues found no difference between recurrence and necrosis groups using 18F-FDG and 11C-MET PET.[173] FDG-PET may have more limited utility than perfusion and DWI in differentiation of tumor progression from radiation necrosis,[176] and although MRS is highly accurate in differentiating between high-grade and low-grade gliomas, it may be less useful in differentiating between true progression and radiation necrosis.[177]

SUMMARY

Treatment response assessment in glioblastoma is important to management decisions and legitimacy of clinical trials. The RANO criteria are the most widely used guidelines in glioma response, but new enhancement seen within the radiation field during the first 12 weeks after treatment is difficult to definitively classify as true progression. Several patterns of enhancement and T2 signal are suggestive of pseudoprogression and radiation necrosis; ultimately, a multimodality approach including advanced imaging has been shown to result in greatest diagnostic accuracy. Pseudoresponse is difficult to discriminate from true response, given that the antiangiogenic effect has been shown to suppress imaging features suggestive of disease progression, even in the absence of increased overall survival. Knowledge of the strengths and limitations of various imaging techniques described previously can help the radiologist to synthesize and integrate provided imaging and clinical data to develop a more evidence-based assessment of true disease progression.

REFERENCES

1. Ostrom QT, Gittleman H, Truitt G, et al. CBTRUS statistical report: primary brain and other central nervous system tumors diagnosed in the United States in 2011–2015. Neuro Oncol 2018; 20(suppl_4):iv1–86.
2. Stupp R, Mason WP, Van Den Bent MJ, et al. Radiotherapy plus concomitant and adjuvant temozolomide for glioblastoma. N Engl J Med 2005; 352(10):987–96.

3. Khasraw M, Ameratunga MS, Grant R, et al. Antiangiogenic therapy for high-grade glioma. Cochrane Database Syst Rev 2014;(9):CD008218.

4. Domingo-Musibay E, Galanis E. What next for newly diagnosed glioblastoma? Future Oncol 2015;11(24):3273–83.

5. Dusek L, Muzik J, Maluskova D, et al. Cancer incidence and mortality in the Czech Republic. Klin Onkol 2014;27(6):406–23.

6. Weathers S-P, Gilbert MR. Current challenges in designing GBM trials for immunotherapy. J Neurooncol 2015;123(3):331–7.

7. Weinberg BD, Gore A, Shu H-KG, et al. Management-based structured reporting of posttreatment glioma response with the brain tumor reporting and data system. J Am Coll Radiol 2018;15(5):767–71.

8. Levin VA, Crafts DC, Norman DM, et al. Criteria for evaluating patients undergoing chemotherapy for malignant brain tumors. J Neurosurg 1977;47(3):329–35.

9. Macdonald DR, Cascino TL, Schold SC Jr, et al. Response criteria for phase II studies of supratentorial malignant glioma. J Clin Oncol 1990;8(7):1277–80.

10. Delgado-Lopez P, Corrales-Garcia E. Survival in glioblastoma: a review on the impact of treatment modalities. Clin Transl Oncol 2016;18(11):1062–71.

11. Eisenhauer EA, Therasse P, Bogaerts J, et al. New response evaluation criteria in solid tumours: revised RECIST guideline (version 1.1). Eur J Cancer 2009;45(2):228–47.

12. Wen PY, Macdonald DR, Reardon DA, et al. Updated response assessment criteria for high-grade gliomas: response assessment in neuro-oncology working group. J Clin Oncol 2010;28(11):1963–72.

13. Okada H, Weller M, Huang R, et al. Immunotherapy response assessment in neuro-oncology: a report of the RANO working group. Lancet Oncol 2015;16(15):e534–42.

14. Okada H, Kohanbash G, Zhu X, et al. Immunotherapeutic approaches for glioma. Crit Rev Immunol 2009;29(1):1–42.

15. Ellingson BM, Wen PY, Cloughesy TF. Modified criteria for radiographic response assessment in glioblastoma clinical trials. Neurotherapeutics 2017;14(2):307–20.

16. Brandsma D, Stalpers L, Taal W, et al. Clinical features, mechanisms, and management of pseudoprogression in malignant gliomas. Lancet Oncol 2008;9(5):453–61.

17. Chaskis C, Neyns B, Michotte A, et al. Pseudoprogression after radiotherapy with concurrent temozolomide for high-grade glioma: clinical observations and working recommendations. Surg Neurol 2009;72(4):423–8.

18. Carceller F, Mandeville H, Mackinnon AD, et al. Facing pseudoprogression after radiotherapy in low grade gliomas. Transl Cancer Res 2017;6(Suppl 2):S254–8.

19. van West SE, de Bruin HG, van de Langerijt B, et al. Incidence of pseudoprogression in low-grade gliomas treated with radiotherapy. Neuro Oncol 2017;19(5):719–25.

20. Clarke JL, Chang S. Pseudoprogression and pseudoresponse: challenges in brain tumor imaging. Curr Neurol Neurosci Rep 2009;9(3):241–6.

21. Dworkin M, Mehan W, Niemierko A, et al. Increase of pseudoprogression and other treatment related effects in low-grade glioma patients treated with proton radiation and temozolomide. J Neurooncol 2019;142(1):69–77.

22. Bronk JK, Guha-Thakurta N, Allen PK, et al. Analysis of pseudoprogression after proton or photon therapy of 99 patients with low grade and anaplastic glioma. Clin Transl Radiat Oncol 2018;9:30–4.

23. De Wit M, De Bruin H, Eijkenboom W, et al. Immediate post-radiotherapy changes in malignant glioma can mimic tumor progression. Neurology 2004;63(3):535–7.

24. Chamberlain MC, Glantz MJ, Chalmers L, et al. Early necrosis following concurrent Temodar and radiotherapy in patients with glioblastoma. J Neurooncol 2007;82(1):81–3.

25. Fatterpekar GM, Galheigo D, Narayana A, et al. Treatment-related change versus tumor recurrence in high-grade gliomas: a diagnostic conundrum—use of dynamic susceptibility contrast-enhanced (DSC) perfusion MRI. AJR Am J Roentgenol 2012;198(1):19–26.

26. Melguizo-Gavilanes I, Bruner JM, Guha-Thakurta N, et al. Characterization of pseudoprogression in patients with glioblastoma: is histology the gold standard? J Neurooncol 2015;123(1):141–50.

27. Weller M, Tabatabai G, Kästner B, et al. MGMT promoter methylation is a strong prognostic biomarker for benefit from dose-intensified temozolomide rechallenge in progressive glioblastoma: the DIRECTOR trial. Clin Cancer Res 2015;21(9):2057–64.

28. Brandes AA, Tosoni A, Franceschi E, et al. Recurrence pattern after temozolomide concomitant with and adjuvant to radiotherapy in newly diagnosed patients with glioblastoma: correlation with MGMT promoter methylation status. J Clin Oncol 2009;27(8):1275–9.

29. Hegi ME, Diserens A-C, Gorlia T, et al. MGMT gene silencing and benefit from temozolomide in glioblastoma. N Engl J Med 2005;352(10):997–1003.

30. Li H, Li J, Cheng G, et al. IDH mutation and MGMT promoter methylation are associated with the pseudoprogression and improved prognosis of

glioblastoma multiforme patients who have under-gone concurrent and adjuvant temozolomide-based chemoradiotherapy. Clin Neurol Neurosurg 2016;151:31–6.

31. Brandes AA, Franceschi E, Tosoni A, et al. MGMT promoter methylation status can predict the inci-dence and outcome of pseudoprogression after concomitant radiochemotherapy in newly diag-nosed glioblastoma patients. J Clin Oncol 2008; 26(13):2192–7.

32. Motegi H, Kamoshima Y, Terasaka S, et al. IDH1 mutation as a potential novel biomarker for distin-guishing pseudoprogression from true progression in patients with glioblastoma treated with temozolo-mide and radiotherapy. Brain Tumor Pathol 2013; 30(2):67–72.

33. Kong D-S, Kim S, Kim E-H, et al. Diagnostic dilemma of pseudoprogression in the treatment of newly diagnosed glioblastomas: the role of assess-ing relative cerebral blood flow volume and oxygen-6-methylguanine-DNA methyltransferase promoter methylation status. AJNR Am J Neurora-diol 2011;32(2):382–7.

34. Drabycz S, Roldán G, De Robles P, et al. An anal-ysis of image texture, tumor location, and MGMT promoter methylation in glioblastoma using mag-netic resonance imaging. Neuroimage 2010;49(2): 1398–405.

35. Yoon RG, Kim HS, Paik W, et al. Different diagnostic values of imaging parameters to predict pseudo-progression in glioblastoma subgroups stratified by MGMT promoter methylation. Eur Radiol 2017; 27(1):255–66.

36. Taal W, Brandsma D, De Bruin H, et al. The incidence of pseudo-progression in a cohort of malignant gli-oma patients treated with chemo-radiation with te-mozolomide. J Clin Oncol 2007;25(18_suppl):2009.

37. van Dijken BR, van Laar PJ, Holtman GA, et al. Diagnostic accuracy of magnetic resonance imag-ing techniques for treatment response evaluation in patients with high-grade glioma, a systematic re-view and meta-analysis. Eur Radiol 2017;27(10): 4129–44.

38. Henegar MM, Moran CJ, Silbergeld DL. Early post-operative magnetic resonance imaging following nonneoplastic cortical resection. J Neurosurg 1996;84(2):174–9.

39. Mullins ME, Barest GD, Schaefer PW, et al. Radia-tion necrosis versus glioma recurrence: conven-tional MR imaging clues to diagnosis. AJNR Am J Neuroradiol 2005;26(8):1967–72.

40. Young R, Gupta A, Shah A, et al. Potential utility of conventional MRI signs in diagnosing pseudoprog-ression in glioblastoma. Neurology 2011;76(22): 1918–24.

41. Yoo R-E, Choi S, Kim T, et al. Independent poor prognostic factors for true progression after

radiation therapy and concomitant temozolomide in patients with glioblastoma: subependymal enhancement and low ADC value. AJNR Am J Neu-roradiol 2015;36(10):1846–52.

42. Reddy K, Westerly D, Chen C. MRI patterns of T 1 enhancing radiation necrosis versus tumour recur-rence in high-grade gliomas. J Med Imaging Ra-diat Oncol 2013;57(3):349–55.

43. Kleinberg L, Yoon G, Weingart JD, et al. Imag-ing after GliaSite brachytherapy: prognostic MRI indicators of disease control and recur-rence. Int J Radiat Oncol Biol Phys 2009;75(5): 1385–91.

44. Dalesandro MF, Andre JB. Posttreatment evalua-tion of brain gliomas. Neuroimage Clin 2016; 26(4):581–99.

45. Abel R, Jones J, Mandelin P, et al. Distinguishing pseudoprogression from true progression by FLAIR volumetric characteristics compared to 45 Gy isodose volumes in treated glioblastoma pa-tients. Int J Radiat Oncol Biol Phys 2012;84(3): S275.

46. Johnson PC, Hunt SJ, Drayer BP. Human cerebral gliomas: correlation of postmortem MR imaging and neuropathologic findings. Radiology 1989; 170(1):211–7.

47. Liu Z-C, Yan L-F, Hu Y-C, et al. Combination of IVIM-DWI and 3D-ASL for differentiating true pro-gression from pseudoprogression of Glioblastoma multiforme after concurrent chemoradiotherapy: study protocol of a prospective diagnostic trial. BMC Med Imaging 2017;17(1):10.

48. Matsusue E, Fink JR, Rockhill JK, et al. Distinction between glioma progression and post-radiation change by combined physiologic MR imaging. Neuroradiology 2010;52(4):297–306.

49. Kim HS, Goh MJ, Kim N, et al. Which combination of MR imaging modalities is best for predicting recurrent glioblastoma? Study of diagnostic accu-racy and reproducibility. Radiology 2014;273(3): 831–43.

50. Cha J, Kim ST, Kim H-J, et al. Differentiation of tu-mor progression from pseudoprogression in pa-tients with posttreatment glioblastoma using multiparametric histogram analysis. AJNR Am J Neuroradiol 2014;35(7):1309–17.

51. Suh CH, Kim HS, Jung SC, et al. Multiparametric MRI as a potential surrogate endpoint for decision-making in early treatment response following concurrent chemoradiotherapy in pa-tients with newly diagnosed glioblastoma: a sys-tematic review and meta-analysis. Eur Radiol 2018;28(6):2628–38.

52. Dickerson E, Srinivasan A. Multicenter survey of current practice patterns in perfusion MRI in neuro-radiology: why, when, and how is it performed? AJR Am J Roentgenol 2016;207(2):406–10.

53. Thust S, Heiland S, Falini A, et al. Glioma imaging in Europe: a survey of 220 centres and recommendations for best clinical practice. Eur Radiol 2018; 28(8):3306–17.

54. Seeger A, Braun C, Skardelly M, et al. Comparison of three different MR perfusion techniques and MR spectroscopy for multiparametric assessment in distinguishing recurrent high-grade gliomas from stable disease. Acad Radiol 2013;20(12):1557–65.

55. McGehee BE, Pollock JM, Maldjian JA. Brain perfusion imaging: how does it work and what should I use? J Magn Reson Imaging 2012;36(6):1257–72.

56. Hu LS, Baxter L, Pinnaduwage D, et al. Optimized preload leakage-correction methods to improve the diagnostic accuracy of dynamic susceptibility-weighted contrast-enhanced perfusion MR imaging in posttreatment gliomas. AJNR Am J Neuroradiol 2010;31(1):40–8.

57. Kelm ZS, Korfiatis PD, Lingineni RK, et al. Variability and accuracy of different software packages for dynamic susceptibility contrast magnetic resonance imaging for distinguishing glioblastoma progression from pseudoprogression. J Med Imaging 2015;2(2):026001.

58. Aronen HJ, Gazit IE, Louis DN, et al. Cerebral blood volume maps of gliomas: comparison with tumor grade and histologic findings. Radiology 1994;191(1):41–51.

59. Sood S, Gupta A, Tsiouris AJ. Advanced magnetic resonance techniques in neuroimaging: diffusion, spectroscopy, and perfusion. Semin Roentgenol 2010;45(2):137–46.

60. Dandois V, Rommel D, Renard L, et al. Substitution of 11C-methionine PET by perfusion MRI during the follow-up of treated high-grade gliomas: preliminary results in clinical practice. J Neuroradiol 2010;37(2):89–97.

61. Di Costanzo A, Scarabino T, Trojsi F, et al. Recurrent glioblastoma multiforme versus radiation injury: a multiparametric 3-T MR approach. Radiol Med 2014;119(8):616–24.

62. Heidemans-Hazelaar C, Van der Kallen B, de Kanter AV, et al. perfusion MR in differentiating between tumor-progression and pseudo-progression in recurrent glioblastoma multiforme: O. 02. Neuro Oncol 2010;12(3):1.

63. Hu LS, Baxter L, Smith K, et al. Relative cerebral blood volume values to differentiate high-grade glioma recurrence from posttreatment radiation effect: direct correlation between image-guided tissue histopathology and localized dynamic susceptibility-weighted contrast-enhanced perfusion MR imaging measurements. AJNR Am J Neuroradiol 2009;30(3):552–8.

64. Mangla R, Singh G, Ziegelitz D, et al. Changes in relative cerebral blood volume 1 month after radiation-temozolomide therapy can help predict overall survival in patients with glioblastoma. Radiology 2010;256(2):575–84.

65. Sugahara T, Korogi Y, Tomiguchi S, et al. Posttherapeutic intraaxial brain tumor: the value of perfusion-sensitive contrast-enhanced MR imaging for differentiating tumor recurrence from nonneoplastic contrast-enhancing tissue. AJNR Am J Neuroradiol 2000;21(5):901–9.

66. Prager A, Martinez N, Beal K, et al. Diffusion and perfusion MRI to differentiate treatment-related changes including pseudoprogression from recurrent tumors in high-grade gliomas with histopathologic evidence. AJNR Am J Neuroradiol 2015; 36(5):877–85.

67. Kerkhof M, Tans PL, Hagenbeek RE, et al. Visual inspection of MR relative cerebral blood volume maps has limited value for distinguishing progression from pseudoprogression in glioblastoma multiforme patients. CNS Oncol 2017;6(04): 297–306.

68. Hyare H, Thust S, Rees J. Advanced MRI techniques in the monitoring of treatment of gliomas. Curr Treat Options Neurol 2017;19(3):11.

69. Patel P, Baradaran H, Delgado D, et al. MR perfusion-weighted imaging in the evaluation of high-grade gliomas after treatment: a systematic review and meta-analysis. Neuro Oncol 2016; 19(1):118–27.

70. Wang Q, Zhang H, Zhang J, et al. The diagnostic performance of magnetic resonance spectroscopy in differentiating high-from low-grade gliomas: a systematic review and meta-analysis. Eur Radiol 2016;26(8):2670–84.

71. Baek HJ, Kim HS, Kim N, et al. Percent change of perfusion skewness and kurtosis: a potential imaging biomarker for early treatment response in patients with newly diagnosed glioblastomas. Radiology 2012;264(3):834–43.

72. Hu LS, Eschbacher JM, Heiserman JE, et al. Reevaluating the imaging definition of tumor progression: perfusion MRI quantifies recurrent glioblastoma tumor fraction, pseudoprogression, and radiation necrosis to predict survival. Neuro Oncol 2012;14(7):919–30.

73. Tsien C, Galbán CJ, Chenevert TL, et al. Parametric response map as an imaging biomarker to distinguish progression from pseudoprogression in high-grade glioma. J Clin Oncol 2010;28(13):2293.

74. Galbán CJ, Chenevert TL, Meyer CR, et al. The parametric response map is an imaging biomarker for early cancer treatment outcome. Nat Med 2009; 15(5):572.

75. Boxerman JL, Ellingson BM, Jeyapalan S, et al. Longitudinal DSC-MRI for distinguishing tumor recurrence from pseudoprogression in patients with a high-grade glioma. Am J Clin Oncol 2017; 40(3):228–34.

76. Paldino MJ, Barboriak DP. Fundamentals of quantitative dynamic contrast-enhanced MR imaging. Magn Reson Imaging Clin N Am 2009;17(2): 277–89.

77. Aquino D, Gioppo A, Finocchiaro G, et al. MRI in glioma immunotherapy: evidence, pitfalls, and perspectives. J Immunol Res 2017;2017:5813951.

78. van Dijken BR, van Laar PJ, Smits M, et al. Perfusion MRI in treatment evaluation of glioblastomas: Clinical relevance of current and future techniques. J Magn Reson Imaging 2019;49(1):11–22.

79. Thomas AA, Arevalo-Perez J, Kaley T, et al. Dynamic contrast enhanced T1 MRI perfusion differentiates pseudoprogression from recurrent glioblastoma. J Neurooncol 2015;125(1):183–90.

80. Bisdas S, Naegele T, Ritz R, et al. Distinguishing recurrent high-grade gliomas from radiation injury: a pilot study using dynamic contrast-enhanced MR imaging. Acad Radiol 2011;18(5):575–83.

81. Yun TJ, Park C-K, Kim TM, et al. Glioblastoma treated with concurrent radiation therapy and temozolomide chemotherapy: differentiation of true progression from pseudoprogression with quantitative dynamic contrast-enhanced MR imaging. Radiology 2015;274(3):830–40.

82. Chung WJ, Kim HS, Kim N, et al. Recurrent glioblastoma: optimum area under the curve method derived from dynamic contrast-enhanced T1-weighted perfusion MR imaging. Radiology 2013; 269(2):561–8.

83. Suh C, Kim H, Choi Y, et al. Prediction of pseudoprogression in patients with glioblastomas using the initial and final area under the curves ratio derived from dynamic contrast-enhanced T1-weighted perfusion MR imaging. AJNR Am J Neuroradiol 2013;34(12):2278–86.

84. Heo YJ, Kim HS, Park JE, et al. Uninterpretable dynamic susceptibility contrast-enhanced perfusion MR images in patients with post-treatment glioblastomas: cross-validation of alternative imaging options. PLoS One 2015;10(8):e0136380.

85. Williams DS, Detre JA, Leigh JS, et al. Magnetic resonance imaging of perfusion using spin inversion of arterial water. Proc Natl Acad Sci U S A 1992;89(1):212–6.

86. Telischak NA, Detre JA, Zaharchuk G. Arterial spin labeling MRI: clinical applications in the brain. J Magn Reson Imaging 2015;41(5):1165–80.

87. Petersen E, Zimine I, Ho YL, et al. Non-invasive measurement of perfusion: a critical review of arterial spin labelling techniques. Br J Radiol 2006; 79(944):688–701.

88. Choi YJ, Kim HS, Jahng G-H, et al. Pseudoprogression in patients with glioblastoma: added value of arterial spin labeling to dynamic susceptibility contrast perfusion MR imaging. Acta Radiol 2013; 54(4):448–54.

89. Schmainda KM. Diffusion-weighted MRI as a biomarker for treatment response in glioma. CNS Oncol 2012;1(2):169–80.

90. Lee WJ, Choi SH, Park C-K, et al. Diffusion-weighted MR imaging for the differentiation of true progression from pseudoprogression following concomitant radiotherapy with temozolomide in patients with newly diagnosed high-grade gliomas. Acad Radiol 2012;19(11):1353–61.

91. Bulik M, Kazda T, Slampa P, et al. The diagnostic ability of follow-up imaging biomarkers after treatment of glioblastoma in the temozolomide era: implications from proton MR spectroscopy and apparent diffusion coefficient mapping. Biomed Res Int 2015;2015:641023.

92. Kazda T, Bulik M, Pospisil P, et al. Advanced MRI increases the diagnostic accuracy of recurrent glioblastoma: single institution thresholds and validation of MR spectroscopy and diffusion weighted MR imaging. Neuroimage Clin 2016;11:316–21.

93. Asao C, Korogi Y, Kitajima M, et al. Diffusion-weighted imaging of radiation-induced brain injury for differentiation from tumor recurrence. AJNR Am J Neuroradiol 2005;26(6):1455–60.

94. Hein PA, Eskey CJ, Dunn JF, et al. Diffusion-weighted imaging in the follow-up of treated high-grade gliomas: tumor recurrence versus radiation injury. AJNR Am J Neuroradiol 2004;25(2):201–9.

95. Reimer C, Deike K, Graf M, et al. Differentiation of pseudoprogression and real progression in glioblastoma using ADC parametric response maps. PLoS One 2017;12(4):e0174620.

96. Gupta A, Young R, Karimi S, et al. Isolated diffusion restriction precedes the development of enhancing tumor in a subset of patients with glioblastoma. AJNR Am J Neuroradiol 2011;32(7):1301–6.

97. Song YS, Choi SH, Park C-K, et al. True progression versus pseudoprogression in the treatment of glioblastomas: a comparison study of normalized cerebral blood volume and apparent diffusion coefficient by histogram analysis. Korean J Radiol 2013;14(4):662–72.

98. Chu HH, Choi SH, Ryoo I, et al. Differentiation of true progression from pseudoprogression in glioblastoma treated with radiation therapy and concomitant temozolomide: comparison study of standard and high-b-value diffusion-weighted imaging. Radiology 2013;269(3):831–40.

99. Nowosielski M, Recheis W, Goebel G, et al. ADC histograms predict response to anti-angiogenic therapy in patients with recurrent high-grade glioma. Neuroradiology 2011;53(4):291–302.

100. Moffat BA, Chenevert TL, Lawrence TS, et al. Functional diffusion map: a noninvasive MRI biomarker for early stratification of clinical brain tumor response. Proc Natl Acad Sci U S A 2005; 102(15):5524–9.

101. Qian X, Tan H, Zhang J, et al. Stratification of pseu-doprogression and true progression of glioblas-toma multiform based on longitudinal diffusion tensor imaging without segmentation. Med Phys 2016;43(11):5889–902.
102. Wang S, Martinez-Lage M, Sakai Y, et al. Differ-entiating tumor progression from pseudoprogres-sion in patients with glioblastomas using diffusion tensor imaging and dynamic susceptibil-ity contrast MRI. AJNR Am J Neuroradiol 2016; 37(1):28–36.
103. Agarwal A, Kumar S, Narang J, et al. Morphologic MRI features, diffusion tensor imaging and radiation dosimetric analysis to differentiate pseudo-progression from early tumor progression. J Neurooncol 2013;112(3):413–20.
104. Sundgren PC, Fan X, Weybright P, et al. Differenti-ation of recurrent brain tumor versus radiation injury using diffusion tensor imaging in patients with new contrast-enhancing lesions. Magn Reson Imaging 2006;24(9):1131–42.
105. Soares D, Law M. Magnetic resonance spectros-copy of the brain: review of metabolites and clinical applications. Clin Radiol 2009;64(1):12–21.
106. Chiang GC, Kovanlikaya I, Choi C, et al. Magnetic resonance spectroscopy, positron emission tomog-raphy and radiogenomics—relevance to glioma. Front Neurol 2018;9:33.
107. Rees J. Diagnosis and treatment in neuro-oncology: an oncological perspective. Br J Radiol 2011;84(special_issue_2):S82–9.
108. Pirzkall A, McKnight TR, Graves EE, et al. MR-spectroscopy guided target delineation for high-grade gliomas. Int J Radiat Oncol Biol Phys 2001; 50(4):915–28.
109. Graves EE, Nelson SJ, Vigneron DB, et al. Serial proton MR spectroscopic imaging of recurrent ma-lignant gliomas after gamma knife radiosurgery. AJNR Am J Neuroradiol 2001;22(4):613–24.
110. Chan AA, Lau A, Pirzkall A, et al. Proton magnetic resonance spectroscopy imaging in the evaluation of patients undergoing gamma knife surgery for Grade IV glioma. J Neurosurg 2004;101(3):467–75.
111. Rock JP, Hearshen D, Scarpace L, et al. Correla-tions between magnetic resonance spectroscopy and image-guided histopathology, with special attention to radiation necrosis. Neurosurgery 2002;51(4):912–20.
112. Lee H, Caparelli E, Li H, et al. Computerized MRS voxel registration and partial volume effects in sin-gle voxel 1H-MRS. Magn Reson Imaging 2013; 31(7):1197–205.
113. Sawlani V, Taylor R, Rowley K, et al. Magnetic resonance spectroscopy for differentiating pseudo-progression from true progression in GBM on concurrent chemoradiotherapy. Neurora-diol J 2012;25(5):575–86.

114. Kaminaga T, Shirai K. Radiation-induced brain metabolic changes in the acute and early delayed phase detected with quantitative proton magnetic resonance spectroscopy. J Comput Assist Tomogr 2005;29(3):293–7.
115. Andronesi OC, Loebel F, Bogner W, et al. Treatment response assessment in IDH-mutant glioma pa-tients by noninvasive 3D functional spectroscopic mapping of 2-hydroxyglutarate. Clin Cancer Res 2016;22(7):1632–41.
116. Choi C, Raisanen JM, Ganji SK, et al. Prospec-tive longitudinal analysis of 2-hydroxyglutarate magnetic resonance spectroscopy identifies broad clinical utility for the management of pa-tients with IDH-mutant glioma. J Clin Oncol 2016;34(33):4030.
117. Brock C, Young H, O'Reilly S, et al. Early evaluation of tumour metabolic response using [18 F] fluoro-deoxyglucose and positron emission tomography: a pilot study following the phase II chemotherapy schedule for temozolomide in recurrent high-grade gliomas. Br J Cancer 2000;82(3):608.
118. Roelcke U, Von Ammon K, Hausmann O, et al. Operated low grade astrocytomas: a long term PET study on the effect of radiotherapy. J Neurol Neurosurg Psychiatry 1999;66(5):644–7.
119. Hölzer T, Herholz K, Jeske J, et al. FDG-PET as a prognostic indicator in radiochemotherapy of glio-blastoma. J Comput Assist Tomogr 1993;17(5): 681–7.
120. Kim E, Chung S, Haynie T, et al. Differentiation of residual or recurrent tumors from post-treatment changes with F-18 FDG PET. Radiographics 1992;12(2):269–79.
121. Wong TZ, Van der Westhuizen GJ, Coleman RE. Positron emission tomography imaging of brain tu-mors. Neuroimage Clin 2002;12(4):615–26.
122. Nihashi T, Dahabreh I, Terasawa T. Diagnostic ac-curacy of PET for recurrent glioma diagnosis: a meta-analysis. AJNR Am J Neuroradiol 2013; 34(5):944–50.
123. Zikou A, Sioka C, Alexiou GA, et al. Radiation ne-crosis, pseudoprogression, pseudoresponse, and tumor recurrence: imaging challenges for the eval-uation of treated gliomas. Contrast Media Mol Im-aging 2018;2018:6828396.
124. Tripathi M, Sharma R, Varshney R, et al. Compari-son of F-18 FDG and C-11 methionine PET/CT for the evaluation of recurrent primary brain tumors. Clin Nucl Med 2012;37(2):158–63.
125. Deuschl C, Kirchner J, Poeppel T, et al. 11 C–MET PET/MRI for detection of recurrent glioma. Eur J Nucl Med Mol Imaging 2018;45(4):593–601.
126. Galldiks N, Dunkl V, Stoffels G, et al. Diagnosis of pseudoprogression in patients with glioblastoma using O-(2-[18 F] fluoroethyl)-L-tyrosine PET. Eur J Nucl Med Mol Imaging 2015;42(5):685–95.

127. Rachinger W, Goetz C, Pöpperl G, et al. Positron emission tomography with O-(2-[18F] fluoroethyl)-l-tyrosine versus magnetic resonance imaging in the diagnosis of recurrent gliomas. Neurosurgery 2005;57(3):505–11.

128. Kebir S, Khurshid Z, Gaertner FC, et al. Unsupervised consensus cluster analysis of [18F]-fluoroethyl-L-tyrosine positron emission tomography identified textural features for the diagnosis of pseudoprogression in high-grade glioma. Oncotarget 2017;8(5):8294.

129. Mehrkens J, Pöpperl G, Rachinger W, et al. The positive predictive value of O-(2-[18 F] fluoroethyl)-L-tyrosine (FET) PET in the diagnosis of a glioma recurrence after multimodal treatment. J Neurooncol 2008;88(1):27–35.

130. Dunet V, Rossier C, Buck A, et al. Performance of 18F-fluoro-ethyl-tyrosine (18F-FET) PET for the differential diagnosis of primary brain tumor: a systematic review and metaanalysis. J Nucl Med 2012;53(2):207–14.

131. Galldiks N, Langen K-J, Pope WB. From the clinician's point of view: what is the status quo of positron emission tomography in patients with brain tumors? Neuro Oncol 2015;17(11):1434–44.

132. Smith MM, Thompson JE, Castillo M, et al. MR of recurrent high-grade astrocytomas after intralesional immunotherapy. AJNR Am J Neuroradiol 1996;17(6):1065–71.

133. Huang RY, Neagu MR, Reardon DA, et al. Pitfalls in the neuroimaging of glioblastoma in the era of antiangiogenic and immuno/targeted therapy–detecting illusive disease, defining response. Front Neurol 2015;6:33.

134. Stenberg L, Englund E, Wirestam R, et al. Dynamic susceptibility contrast-enhanced perfusion magnetic resonance (MR) imaging combined with contrast-enhanced MR imaging in the follow-up of immunogene-treated glioblastoma multiforme. Acta Radiol 2006;47(8):852–61.

135. Vrabec M, Van Cauter S, Himmelreich U, et al. MR perfusion and diffusion imaging in the follow-up of recurrent glioblastoma treated with dendritic cell immunotherapy: a pilot study. Neuroradiology 2011;53(10):721–31.

136. Qin L, Li X, Stroiney A, et al. Advanced MRI assessment to predict benefit of anti-programmed cell death 1 protein immunotherapy response in patients with recurrent glioblastoma. Neuroradiology 2017;59(2):135–45.

137. Floeth F, Wittsack H-J, Engelbrecht V, et al. Comparative follow-up of enhancement phenomena with MRI and proton MR spectroscopic imaging after intralesional immunotherapy in glioblastoma. Zentralbl Neurochir 2002;63(01):23–8.

138. Pellegatta S, Eoli M, Frigerio S, et al. The natural killer cell response and tumor debulking are associated with prolonged survival in recurrent glioblastoma patients receiving dendritic cells loaded with autologous tumor lysates. Oncoimmunology 2013;2(3):e23401.

139. Wang N, Jain RK, Batchelor TT. New directions in anti-angiogenic therapy for glioblastoma. Neurotherapeutics 2017;14(2):321–32.

140. Jain RK, Di Tomaso E, Duda DG, et al. Angiogenesis in brain tumours. Nat Rev Neurosci 2007;8(8):610.

141. Batchelor TT, Sorensen AG, di Tomaso E, et al. AZD2171, a pan-VEGF receptor tyrosine kinase inhibitor, normalizes tumor vasculature and alleviates edema in glioblastoma patients. Cancer Cell 2007;11(1):83–95.

142. Friedman HS, Prados MD, Wen PY, et al. Bevacizumab alone and in combination with irinotecan in recurrent glioblastoma. J Clin Oncol 2009;27(28):4733–40.

143. Norden A, Young G, Setayesh K, et al. Bevacizumab for recurrent malignant gliomas. Efficacy, toxicity, and patterns of recurrence. Neurology 2008;70(10):779–87.

144. Boxerman JL, Zhang Z, Safriel Y, et al. Prognostic value of contrast enhancement and FLAIR for survival in newly diagnosed glioblastoma treated with and without bevacizumab: results from ACRIN 6686. Neuro Oncol 2018;20(10):1400–10.

145. Stadlbauer A, Pichler P, Karl M, et al. Quantification of serial changes in cerebral blood volume and metabolism in patients with recurrent glioblastoma undergoing antiangiogenic therapy. Eur J Radiol 2015;84(6):1128–36.

146. Sorensen AG, Emblem KE, Polaskova P, et al. Increased survival of glioblastoma patients who respond to antiangiogenic therapy with elevated blood perfusion. Cancer Res 2012;72(2):402–7.

147. Hilario A, Sepulveda J, Hernandez-Lain A, et al. Leakage decrease detected by dynamic susceptibility-weighted contrast-enhanced perfusion MRI predicts survival in recurrent glioblastoma treated with bevacizumab. Clin Transl Oncol 2017;19(1):51–7.

148. Auer TA, Breit H-C, Marini F, et al. Evaluation of the apparent diffusion coefficient in patients with recurrent glioblastoma under treatment with bevacizumab with radiographic pseudoresponse. J Neuroradiol 2019;46(1):36–43.

149. Ellingson BM, Gerstner ER, Smits M, et al. Diffusion MRI phenotypes predict overall survival benefit from anti-VEGF monotherapy in recurrent glioblastoma: converging evidence from phase II trials. Clin Cancer Res 2017;23(19):5745–56.

150. Galldiks N, Rapp M, Stoffels G, et al. Earlier diagnosis of progressive disease during bevacizumab treatment using O-(2-18F-fluorethyl)-L-tyrosine positron emission tomography in comparison with

magnetic resonance imaging. Mol Imaging 2013; 12(5):273–6.

151. Schwarzenberg J, Czernin J, Cloughesy TF, et al. Treatment response evaluation using 18F-FDOPA PET in patients with recurrent malignant glioma on bevacizumab therapy. Clin Cancer Res 2014; 20(13):3550–9.

152. Alexiou GA, Zikou A, Tsiouris S, et al. Comparison of diffusion tensor, dynamic susceptibility contrast MRI and 99mTc-Tetrofosmin brain SPECT for the detection of recurrent high-grade glioma. Magn Reson Imaging 2014;32(7):854–9.

153. Gasparetto EL, Pawlak MA, Patel SH, et al. Post-treatment recurrence of malignant brain neoplasm: accuracy of relative cerebral blood volume fraction in discriminating low from high malignant histologic volume fraction. Radiology 2009;250(3):887–96.

154. Narang J, Jain R, Arbab AS, et al. Differentiating treatment-induced necrosis from recurrent/progressive brain tumor using nonmodel-based semiquantitative indices derived from dynamic contrast-enhanced T1-weighted MR perfusion. Neuro Oncol 2011;13(9):1037–46.

155. Rahmathulla G, Marko NF, Weil RJ. Cerebral radiation necrosis: a review of the pathobiology, diagnosis and management considerations. J Clin Neurosci 2013;20(4):485–502.

156. Marks JE, Bagĺan RJ, Prassad SC, et al. Cerebral radionecrosis: incidence and risk in relation to dose, time, fractionation and volume. Int J Radiat Oncol Biol Phys 1981;7(2):243–52.

157. Acharya S, Robinson CG, Michalski JM, et al. Association of 1p/19q codeletion and radiation necrosis in adult cranial gliomas after proton or photon therapy. Int J Radiat Oncol Biol Phys 2018;101(2): 334–43.

158. Kumar AJ, Leeds NE, Fuller GN, et al. Malignant gliomas: MR imaging spectrum of radiation therapy-and chemotherapy-induced necrosis of the brain after treatment. Radiology 2000;217(2): 377–84.

159. Aiken AH, Chang SM, Larson D, et al. Longitudinal magnetic resonance imaging features of glioblastoma multiforme treated with radiotherapy with or without brachytherapy. Int J Radiat Oncol Biol Phys 2008;72(5):1340–6.

160. Ryken TC, Aygun N, Morris J, et al. The role of imaging in the management of progressive glioblastoma. J Neurooncol 2014;118(3):435–60.

161. Al Sayyari A, Buckley R, McHenery C, et al. Distinguishing recurrent primary brain tumor from radiation injury: a preliminary study using a susceptibility-weighted MR imaging– guided apparent diffusion coefficient analysis strategy. AJNR Am J Neuroradiol 2010;31(6):1049–54.

162. Ringelstein A, Turowski B, Gizewski E, et al. Evaluation of ADC mapping as an early predictor for

163. Pica A, Hauf M, Slotboom J, et al. P. 074* dynamic susceptibility contrast perfusion MRI in differentiating radiation necrosis from tumor recurrence in high-grade gliomas. Neuro Oncol 2012;14(suppl_3):iii1–94.

164. Barajas RF Jr, Chang JS, Segal MR, et al. Differentiation of recurrent glioblastoma multiforme from radiation necrosis after external beam radiation therapy with dynamic susceptibility-weighted contrast-enhanced perfusion MR imaging. Radiology 2009;253(2):486–96.

165. Larsen VA, Simonsen HJ, Law I, et al. Evaluation of dynamic contrast-enhanced T1-weighted perfusion MRI in the differentiation of tumor recurrence from radiation necrosis. Neuroradiology 2013; 55(3):361–9.

166. Ozsunar Y, Mullins ME, Kwong K, et al. Glioma recurrence versus radiation necrosis? A pilot comparison of arterial spin-labeled, dynamic susceptibility contrast enhanced MRI, and FDG-PET imaging. Acad Radiol 2010;17(3):282–90.

167. Srinivasan R, Phillips JJ, VandenBerg SR, et al. Ex vivo MR spectroscopic measure differentiates tumor from treatment effects in GBM. Neuro Oncol 2010;12(11):1152–61.

168. Weybright P, Sundgren PC, Maly P, et al. Differentiation between brain tumor recurrence and radiation injury using MR spectroscopy. AJR Am J Roentgenol 2005;185(6):1471–6.

169. Rabinov JD, Lee PL, Barker FG, et al. In vivo 3-T MR spectroscopy in the distinction of recurrent glioma versus radiation effects: initial experience. Radiology 2002;225(3):871–9.

170. Wald LL, Nelson SJ, Day MR, et al. Serial proton magnetic resonance spectroscopy imaging of glioblastoma multiforme after brachytherapy. J Neurosurg 1997;87(4):525–34.

171. Enslow MS, Zollinger LV, Morton KA, et al. Comparison of F-18 fluorodeoxyglucose and F-18 fluorothymidine positron emission tomography in differentiating radiation necrosis from recurrent glioma. Clin Nucl Med 2012;37(9):854.

172. Rollin N, Guyotat J, Streichenberger N, et al. Clinical relevance of diffusion and perfusion magnetic resonance imaging in assessing intra-axial brain tumors. Neuroradiology 2006;48(3): 150–9.

173. Kim YH, Oh SW, Lim YJ, et al. Differentiating radiation necrosis from tumor recurrence in high-grade gliomas: assessing the efficacy of 18F-FDG PET, 11C-methionine PET and perfusion MRI. Clin Neurol Neurosurg 2010;112(9):758–65.

174. Chernov M, Hayashi M, Izawa M, et al. Differentiation of the radiation-induced necrosis and tumor

recurrence after gamma knife radiosurgery for brain metastases: importance of multi-voxel proton MRS. Minim Invasive Neurosurg 2005;48(04): 228–34.

175. Zhang H, Ma L, Wang Q, et al. Role of magnetic resonance spectroscopy for the differentiation of recurrent glioma from radiation necrosis: a systematic review and meta-analysis. Eur J Radiol 2014; 83(12):2181–9.

176. Pötzi C, Becherer A, Marosi C, et al. [11C] methionine and [18F] fluorodeoxyglucose PET in the follow-up of glioblastoma multiforme. J Neurooncol 2007;84(3):305.

177. Hollingworth W, Medina L, Lenkinski R, et al. A systematic literature review of magnetic resonance spectroscopy for the characterization of brain tumors. AJNR Am J Neuroradiol 2006;27(7): 1404–11.

Central Nervous System Lesions in Immunocompromised Patients

Robert Y. Shih, MD[a],*, Kelly K. Koeller, MD[b],[1]

KEYWORDS

- CNS • Immunodeficiency • Infection • PCNSL • EBV-SMT

KEY POINTS

- Immunodeficiency may affect different components of the immune system (physical barriers, neutrophils, humoral, and cellular) and predispose to different types of opportunistic infections.
- HIV/AIDS and immunosuppressive therapy for organ transplantation or autoimmune disease impair cellular immunity (T-cell deficiency) and increase the risk from intracellular pathogens.
- The most frequent central nervous system (CNS) opportunistic infections in HIV/AIDS are tuberculosis (bacteria), cryptococcosis (fungus), toxoplasmosis (parasite), and progressive multifocal leukoencephalopathy (virus).
- Both clinical and radiologic signs of an inflammatory response (eg, fever and enhancement) may decrease in the setting of immunodeficiency and increase with immune reconstitution.
- Differential diagnosis for enhancing parenchymal or dural masses in an immunocompromised patient should include CNS lymphoma or Epstein-Barr virus–associated smooth muscle tumor, respectively.

INTRODUCTION

The innate and adaptive immune systems are responsible for defending bodies through a continuous process of detecting and destroying foreign or abnormal cells. The innate immune system is the more basic or nonspecific and is present in most multicellular organisms, including plants, fungi, and insects. It is composed of physical barriers (eg, skin or mucosa), humoral components (eg, complement or cytokines), and cellular components (eg, phagocytes or natural killer cells). In contrast, the adaptive or acquired immune system is a much more recent evolutionary development (approximately 500 million years ago), unique to higher jawed vertebrates.[1] It has both humoral (eg, antibodies) and cellular (eg, lymphocytes) components. Among B lymphocytes and T lymphocytes, recombination-activating genes gave rise to rearranging antigen-binding receptors that

Disclaimer: The views expressed in this article are those of the authors and do not reflect the official policy of the Department of Defense or US Government.

Disclosure of Conflicts of Interest: K.K. Koeller: Activities related to the present article: consulting agreement with Mayo Clinic to provide support, as the Section Chief of Neuroradiology, for the American Institute for Radiologic Pathology, a program of the American College of Radiology. Activities not related to the present article: consulting agreement with Mayo Clinic to provide support, as the Section Chief of Neuroradiology, for the American Institute for Radiologic Pathology, a program of the American College of Radiology. Other activities: disclosed no relevant relationships.

[a] Department of Radiology, Uniformed Services University, 4301 Jones Bridge Road, Bethesda, MD 20814, USA;
[b] Department of Radiology, Mayo Clinic Minnesota, 200 First Street Southwest, Rochester, MN 55905, USA
[1] Senior author.
* Corresponding author.
E-mail address: robert.shih@usuhs.edu

Radiol Clin N Am 57 (2019) 1217–1231
https://doi.org/10.1016/j.rcl.2019.07.002
0033-8389/19/Published by Elsevier Inc.

permit a few hundred genes to specifically recognize and thereby adapt to millions of potential antigens.

From a broad point of view, a defect in any of these host defenses may be considered an immunodeficiency, including a disruption of physical barriers (eg, craniotomy and ventriculostomy). Primary or genetic immunodeficiency is less frequent than secondary or acquired immunodeficiency; either may affect different components of the immune system and, therefore, predispose to different types of opportunistic infections.[2,3] For example, a defect in neutrophil function or humoral immunity increases risk from disseminated infection by extracellular pathogens (eg, bacterial or fungal sepsis), whereas a defect in cytotoxic activity by natural killer cells or $CD8^+$ T lymphocytes increases risk from intracellular pathogens (eg, mycobacteria or viruses). Because $CD4^+$ T lymphocytes play a significant role in stimulating and regulating both humoral and cellular immune responses, T-cell deficiency underlies many of the secondary causes that result in immunocompromised patients.

These secondary or acquired causes include cancer (eg, chemotherapy), human immunodeficiency virus (HIV) (eg, AIDS), and immunosuppressive therapy (eg, glucocorticoids). In response to the events of 9/11 and subsequent anthrax attacks, an analysis from 2002 on the theoretic risks of mass smallpox vaccination estimated as many as 10 million immunocompromised persons in the United States (3.6% of the population).[4] These individuals will have elevated susceptibility not only to infections but also to tumors, due to impaired immune surveillance for transformed cells by cytotoxic lymphocytes. The inverse of this principle, the enhancement of T lymphocyte activity against cancer by the inhibition of cellular brakes like CTLA-4 and PD-1, was the basis for awarding the 2018 Nobel Prize in Physiology or Medicine to James Allison and Tasuku Honjo.[5] The purpose of this article is to discuss central nervous system (CNS) lesions—infectious (bacterial, fungal, parasitic, and viral) and neoplastic—that may be seen in the setting of immunodeficiency (Table 1).

BACTERIAL LESIONS

Bacteria are prokaryotic microorganisms, lacking nuclei or membrane-bound organelles, that first appeared on planet Earth approximately 4 billion years ago. As potential agents of infectious diseases, they can be roughly subdivided into pyogenic bacteria, which tend to present acutely with a strong neutrophilic response (suppuration), and atypical bacteria, which tend to evade first responders and present less acutely with a

Table 1
Five categories of central nervous system lesions in immunocompromised patients (overview of common features)

Category	Disease	Meninges	Parenchyma	Laboratory
Bacterial	Tuberculosis	Meningitis	Tuberculomas	CSF PCR/culture
	Nocardiosis	Meningitis	Brain abscess	Brain/lung biopsy
Fungal	Cryptococcosis	Meningitis	Gelatinous pseudocysts	CrAg in serum or CSF, CSF culture
	Candidiasis	Meningitis	Microabscesses	Blood culture
	Aspergillosis		Abscess, infarcts	Sputum culture
	Mucormycosis	Invasion from rhinosinusitis	Invasion from rhinosinusitis	Sinonasal biopsy
Parasitic	Toxoplasmosis		Ring-enhancing lesions	CSF Ab, CSF PCR, empiric therapy
	Acanthamoebiasis		Necrosis and hemorrhage	Brain biopsy
Viral	HIV		Chronic white matter gliosis	HIV viral levels
	PML		Demyelinating lesions	CSF PCR, biopsy is gold standard
	CMV		Ventriculoencephalitis	CSF viral levels
Neoplastic	PCNSL		Ring-enhancing lesions	CSF EBV PCR, CSF cytology, biopsy
	EBV-SMT	Dural-based masses		CSF EBV PCR, biopsy

Abbreviations: Ab, antibody; CrAg, cryptococcal antigen.

macrophage-centered response (granulomas).[6] Acute pyogenic bacterial meningitis may cause fever, neck stiffness, and/or altered mental status in immunocompetent patients; because most common etiologies (*Streptococcus pneumoniae*, *Neisseria meningitidis*, and *Haemophilus influenzae*) possess protective polysaccharide capsules, immunocompromised patients with antibody or humoral immune system defects are particularly susceptible, whether they arise from primary/genetic reasons (eg, X-linked agammaglobulinemia) or secondary/acquired ones (eg, splenic injury).[7–9]

When acute bacterial meningitis is suspected, rapid initiation of empiric antimicrobial therapy after blood cultures (before head computed tomography [CT] or lumbar puncture) is recommended to reduce morbidity and mortality. In patients with impaired cellular immunity, including at extremes of age (<1 month or >50 years), antibiotic coverage should be broadened to include *Listeria monocytogenes* and gram-negative bacilli.[10] Meningitis is a clinical and laboratory diagnosis.

Although neuroimaging may reveal thin signal abnormality or enhancement in the cerebral sulci, it also may be normal and is most useful to look for secondary findings, such as parenchymal involvement. In 1983, Enzmann and colleagues[11] used serial contrast-enhanced CT to describe 4 stages of abscess development: early cerebritis (ill-defined hypodensity), late cerebritis (ill-defined ring enhancement), early capsule, and late capsule (well-defined enhancing rim). In 1980, they observed this process is attenuated in the immunocompromised.[12]

Listeria is a genus of gram-positive rods, named after the pioneer of sterile surgery Sir Joseph Lister. *L monocytogenes*, a foodborne pathogen, may cause a self-limited febrile gastroenteritis. Because of its ability to escape the phagosome and hide intracellularly within macrophages, it can also cause invasive listeriosis, typically in patients with varying degrees of T-cell deficiency (eg, neonates or elderly; pregnancy, especially third-trimester; cancer; AIDS; organ transplant;

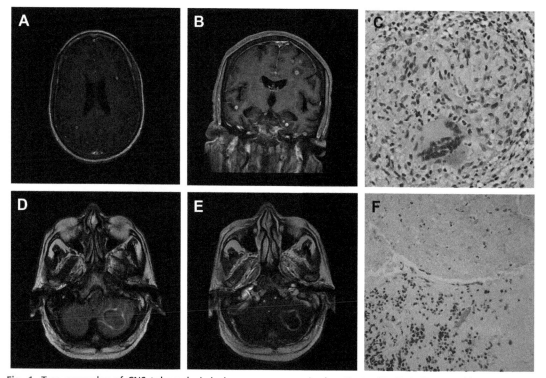

Fig. 1. Two examples of CNS tuberculosis in immunocompromised patients. (*A*, *B*) A 61-year-old woman with AIDS, tuberculous meningitis (diagnosed by CSF), and small enhancing parenchymal tuberculomas on axial and coronal postcontrast T1-weighted images. (*C*) Hematoxylin-eosin stain photomicrograph of a tuberculoma shows a rounded collection of epithelioid macrophages with a multinucleated giant cell at the bottom. (*D*, *E*) A 71-year-old man status post renal transplant with a ring-enhancing left cerebellar tuberculous abscess on axial T2-weighted FLAIR and postcontrast T1-weighted images, which underwent surgical biopsy and drainage. (*F*) Hematoxylin-eosin stain photomicrograph shows purulent debris at the top and vascularized abscess wall with inflammatory cells at the bottom. Tuberculous abscesses are less common than tuberculomas and usually are seen in the immunocompromised. ([*A*, *B*] *Courtesy of* Dr. Stephanie George and MedPix®; with permission.)

and glucocorticoid therapy).[13,14] Spread through the bloodstream and seeding of the CNS may result in meningitis (which may progress to meningoencephalitis) or cerebritis (which may progress to abscess formation). On imaging, this can manifest as T2 signal abnormality or pathologic enhancement in the cerebrospinal fluid (CSF) spaces or brain parenchyma, respectively. *Listeria* is the most common cause of rhombencephalitis, specifically inflammation of the hindbrain (brainstem/cerebellum); however, all these findings remain nonspecific.[15,16]

Atypical bacterial infections tend to evade the acute inflammatory response. They include both intracellular (eg, mycobacteria) and extracellular (eg, spirochetes) pathogens, which may cause disease in either immunocompetent or immunocompromised patients. For example, both tuberculosis and syphilis can produce a thick enhancing meningitis with predilection for the basal cisterns and secondary arteritis; they also can deposit enhancing granulomas within the brain parenchyma (tuberculomas or gummas).[6]

Tuberculomas may demonstrate solid or ringlike enhancement, depending on the amount of caseating necrosis; thus, there is some overlap in appearance with rare ring-enhancing tuberculous brain abscess, although the latter presents with a more rapidly deteriorating clinical course (**Fig. 1**).[17] *Nocardia*, similar to *Mycobacterium tuberculosis* with a moldlike growth pattern and mycolic acids in the cell wall, can also spread from the lungs to the CNS (usually in immunocompromised patients) and may cause meningitis, granuloma, or abscess.[18] *Mycobacterium* (Greek: *myco* = fungus) and *Nocardia* are both genera in the order *Actinomycetales*; actinomycetes are bacteria that were once classified as fungi.

FUNGAL LESIONS

In contrast to bacteria, fungi are eukaryotes with nuclei and other membrane-bound organelles. Compared with other eukaryotes, they are genetically more closely related to animals than to plants. Like animals, fungi are unable to make their

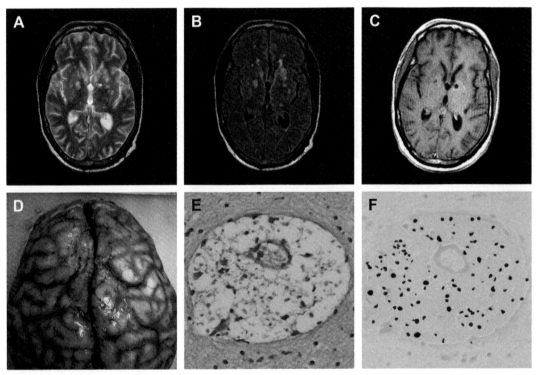

Fig. 2. A 39-year-old man with diplopia, headache, and altered mental status who decompensated after intensive care unit admission; autopsy revealed unsuspected HIV infection with disseminated cryptococcosis. (*A–C*) Axial T2-weighted, T2-weighted FLAIR, and postcontrast T1-weighted images reveal nonenhancing T2/FLAIR hyperintense gelatinous pseudocysts in the bilateral basal ganglia. (*D*) Gross photograph shows thickened leptomeninges from cryptococcal meningitis. (*E, F*) Hematoxylin-eosin stain and Grocott methenamine silver stain photomicrographs show a small vessel at the top center and a soap bubble dilated perivascular space with fungal organisms (appear black on Grocott methenamine silver stain). This is the pathologic correlate of gelatinous pseudocysts.

own food (heterotrophs) and can be structured as unicellular or multicellular organisms. Unicellular yeasts include *Saccharomyces cerevisiae*, used in the brewing of ale or the baking of bread; yeast pathogens include *Cryptococcus* and *Candida* species. Multicellular molds demonstrate a filamentous/hyphal growth pattern and reproduce via spore production; mold pathogens include *Aspergillus* and *Mucorales* species. A third category grows as mold at room temperature and yeast or spherules at body temperature (dimorphic fungi); example pathogens include *Blastomyces dermatitidis*, *Coccidioides immitis*, and *Histoplasma capsulatum*.[6]

Cryptococcus is an encapsulated yeast found in bird or mammal droppings; cryptococcosis is the most common fungal infection of the CNS and initially involves the lungs after basidiospore inhalation.[19] Most cases result from *C neoformans* and occur in immunocompromised patients, although *C gattii* is a rare cause of disseminated

infection in immunocompetent patients. Meningitis can be imaging negative or can show expanded soap bubble perivascular spaces (capsular material or gelatinous pseudocysts) (**Fig. 2**). Parenchymal granulomas (cryptococcomas) are less common and may be nonenhancing in the setting of impaired immune function.[20,21] Diagnosis is established by lumbar puncture and CSF culture. *Candida* is another small yeast that can access the microcirculation and cause meningitis or parenchymal disease in immunocompromised patients, usually in the setting of known fungemia (*C albicans*). Microabscesses less than 3 mm, which may be hemorrhagic due to pseudohyphal invasion, are characteristic.[20,22]

Aspergillus (usually *A fumigatus*) is a mold with septate branching hyphae that causes invasive disease in immunocompromised patients, especially on chronic immunosuppressive therapy (eg, solid organ transplant recipient) or after allogenic stem cell transplantation for hematologic

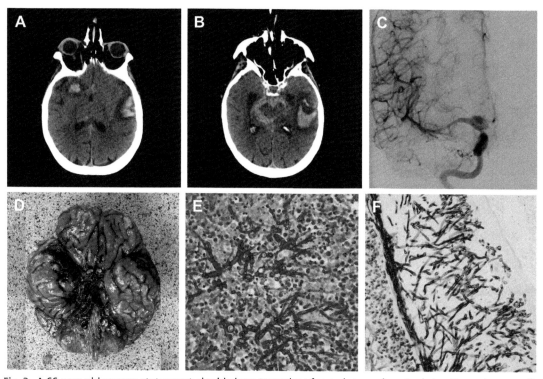

Fig. 3. A 66-year-old woman status post–double lung transplant for end-stage chronic obstructive pulmonary disease with new seizures. (*A, B*) Head CT images reveal multiple peripheral parenchymal hemorrhages and subarachnoid blood in the perimesencephalic cisterns due to hematogenous dissemination of angioinvasive aspergillosis. (*C*) Cerebral angiography (right internal carotid artery injection) depicts a mycotic pseudoaneurysm of the right A1 segment. (*D*) Gross photograph confirms subarachnoid blood along the undersurface of the right frontotemporal lobes. (*E*) Hematoxylin-eosin stain photomicrograph shows dichotomous (approximately 45°) branching of septate hyphae, consistent with *Aspergillus* species. (*F*) Grocott methenamine silver stain photomicrograph demonstrates fungal hyphae invading a vessel wall (compare filamentous appearance vs unicellular yeast of *Cryptococcus*).

cancer.[23,24] The multicellular hyphae are too large to seed the meningeal microcirculation; instead they directly invade the brain or vessels from the bloodstream, causing parenchymal abscesses or infarction/hemorrhages, respectively (**Fig. 3**).[20,25] Like other abscesses, diffusion-weighted imaging is useful for identifying pus, whose cellular debris and high viscosity restrict the motion of water molecules. Peripheral enhancement may be weak or absent in patients unable to mount an inflammatory response.[26] Filamentous fungi in the order *Mucorales* can also invade brain/vessels in immunocompromised patients, usually via extension from rhinosinusitis (rhinocerebral mucormycosis) not hematogenous dissemination (**Fig. 4**).[20,27] *Aspergillus* is also capable of causing invasive fungal sinusitis and rhinocerebral disease, with typical involvement of the adjacent orbits, inferior frontal lobes, or basal ganglia and with characteristic hyperattenuation or T2 hypointensity of

accumulated fungal elements due to increased protein content.

Most of the previously described fungi are ubiquitous in the environment and are pathogenic under immunodeficient conditions. Dimorphic fungi (also known as endemic fungi) are localized to geographic distributions and may cause disease in the immunocompetent or immunocompromised. *C immitis* is the most likely to involve the CNS (via dissemination from the lungs after inhalation of dust containing spores) and is endemic to the southwestern United States and northern Mexico. Abnormal leptomeningeal enhancement in the basal cisterns and spinal canal is the most common imaging finding for CNS coccidioidomycosis. Similar to tuberculous meningitis, it may result in hydrocephalus or vascular complications (infarcts or hemorrhages) and parenchymal granulomas (coccidioidomycomas), which are rare.[28] Disseminated *B dermatitidis* (blastomycosis) and

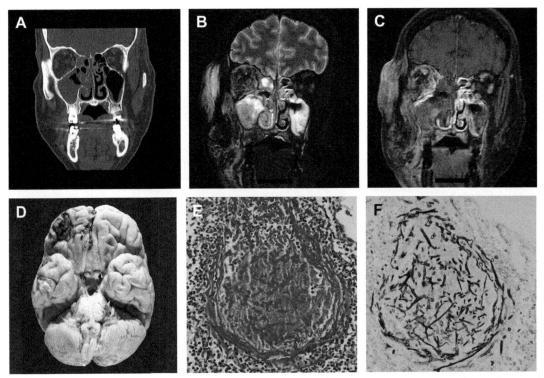

Fig. 4. A 43-year old man with acute myeloid leukemia and neutropenia status post 3 cycles of cytarabine and idarubicin had right eye then face pain and fevers for 5 days. (*A*) Coronally reformatted sinus CT image illustrates near complete opacification of the right nasal cavity and maxillary/ethmoid sinuses. (*B, C*) Coronal T2-weighted and postcontrast T1-weighted images with fat saturation characterize the opacification as heterogeneously T2 hyperintense and nonenhancing. Loss of nasal mucosa enhancement is known as the black turbinate sign and is consistent with angioinvasive mucormycosis. MR imaging also reveals invasion of the right medial orbit and right gyrus rectus (also known as rhinocerebral mucormycosis). (*D*) Gross photograph shows blood along the right inferior frontal lobe. (*E, F*) Hematoxylin-eosin stain and Grocott methenamine silver stain photomicrographs depict numerous fungal elements within the lumen and wall of a small cerebral blood vessel. These hyphae are aseptate and branch at approximately 90° angles, which is consistent with *Mucorales* species.

H capsulatum (histoplasmosis) also can produce a neuroimaging pattern of meningitis or parenchymal granulomas[20] (**Fig. 5**).

PARASITIC LESIONS

A parasite is an organism that lives on or in another organism and that also benefits from this relationship at the other's expense, which is true of most infectious pathogens. Protozoa (Greek: *protos zoion* = first animal) are mobile unicellular eukaryotes without capability for photosynthesis and include parasitic CNS pathogens. Although mobile multicellular eukaryotic heterotrophic parasites (ie, worms) also can infect the CNS (eg, neurocysticercosis and schistosomiasis), they are not considered opportunistic infections, and, in some cases, the lack of a host immune response to the cysticerci of *Taenia solium* or the eggs of *Schistosoma japonicum* may actually help protect against the development of neurologic symptoms.[29]

The most important parasitic opportunistic infection of the CNS is toxoplasmosis, which is also the most common cause of cerebral abscesses in HIV/AIDS (especially CD4 count <100 cells/mm^3); the incidence dropped markedly with introduction of highly active antiretroviral therapy (HAART) in 1996.[19,30] *Toxoplasma gondii* is an obligate intracellular protozoan, whose definitive hosts are felines. Humans and other warmblooded animals can become intermediate hosts by fecal-oral transmission of oocysts containing sporozoites from infected definitive hosts (cat excrement) or by ingestion/transplantation of tissue cysts containing bradyzoites from other intermediate hosts (brain/muscle).[31] This tropism for the CNS has been shown to modify rodent behavior such that they are more likely to be consumed by feline predators and perpetuate the parasite's lifecycle; some studies have linked infection to schizophrenia or poor impulse regulation in humans.[32] Primary and latent infections are usually asymptomatic; exposure or reactivation in

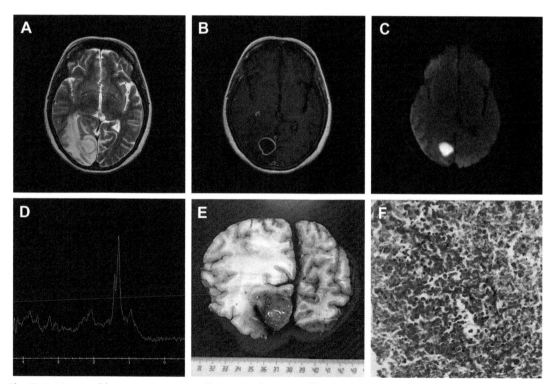

Fig. 5. A 44-year-old woman status post liver transplantation (for autoimmune cirrhosis) on prednisone and tacrolimus with new headache and vomiting. (*A, B*) Axial T2-weighted and postcontrast T1-weighted images reveal a ring-enhancing lesion in the right occipital lobe with extensive vasogenic edema. (*C*) Axial DWI shows central restricted diffusion, which suggests highly viscous contents. The differential diagnosis includes pyogenic, tuberculous, and fungal abscesses. (*D*) MR spectroscopy (echo time 35 ms) identifies elevated lactate and lipid peaks at 0.9 ppm to 1.4 ppm, which is a nonspecific finding. (*E*) Gross photograph shows a round encapsulated lesion with greenish-yellow contents. (*F*) Hematoxylin-eosin stain photomicrograph depicts necroinflammatory debris with pigmented septate hyphae and yeastlike structures (chromoblastomycosis).

an immunocompromised patient may cause toxoplasmic encephalitis. The most classic imaging pattern is multiple ring-enhancing cerebral abscesses with predilection for the basal ganglia. An enhancing nodule (eccentric target sign) is highly specific but seen in less than 30% of cases (**Fig. 6**).[33,34]

Chagas disease is another example of a chronic infection by a protozoan parasite that is able to reactivate in the immunocompromised patient (eg, HIV/AIDS or immunosuppressive medications). Also known as (Latin) American trypanosomiasis, it is caused by *Trypanosoma cruzi*, which is transmitted to humans (definitive host) from triatomine bugs (intermediate host). These kissing bugs preferentially bite the face for their blood meal, when they can also defecate and deposit infectious trypomastigotes. Like toxoplasmosis, alternative routes of transmission include blood transfusions, organ transplantation, and transplacental from mother to child. Unlike toxoplasmosis, acute or chronic Chagas disease may be

symptomatic in the immunocompetent patient (eg, Romaña sign or cardiomyopathy). With regard to the CNS, meningoencephalitis can be seen in both immunocompetent and immunocompromised, whereas brain abscess or mass lesions (chagomas) are seen only in the immunocompromised (**Fig. 7**).[29]

The colorful phrase, brain-eating ameba, refers to *Naegleria fowleri*, a protozoan that lives warm freshwater and enters the nose to cause primary amebic encephalitis in the immunocompetent. In contrast, granulomatous amebic encephalitis usually affects the immunocompromised and is caused by *Acanthamoeba* species (acanthamoebiasis). These free-living amebae are found in soil and can infect the skin or lower respiratory tract before hematogenous spread to the CNS. There, they cause a subacute-to-chronic granulomatous inflammation with necrosis/hemorrhage from thrombotic angiitis. On imaging, the most common presentation is multifocal parenchymal edema (sometimes unifocal early in the disease course)

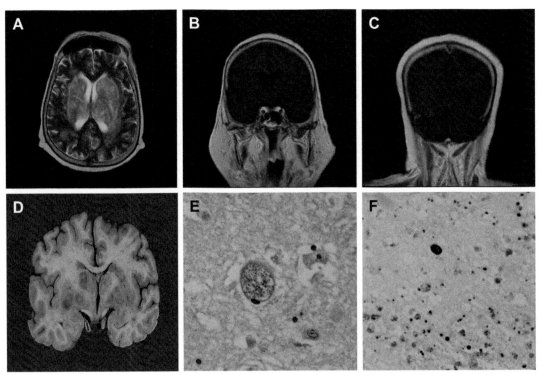

Fig. 6. A 63-year-old woman on rituximab for recent diagnosis of idiopathic thrombocytopenia purpura with altered mental status. (*A*) Axial T2-weighted image demonstrates multiple T2 hyperintense lesions in the bilateral basal ganglia and cerebral hemispheres. (*B, C*) Coronal postcontrast T1-weighted images show small subtle enhancing foci in the bilateral basal ganglia and near the gray-white matter interface, consistent with hematogenous dissemination. Some of the larger occipital lesions are ring enhancing. (*D*) Gross photograph with multiple round tan lesions in the basal ganglia. (*E*) Hematoxylin-eosin stain photomicrograph depicts a toxoplasma tissue cyst (containing bradyzoites) in the center of the image. (*F*) An immunohistochemical stain for *T gondii* highlights both the tissue cysts (*larger*) and free tachyzoites (*smaller*).

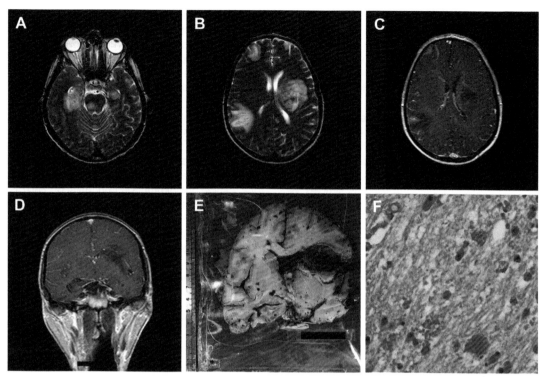

Fig. 7. A 56-year-old man with recent renal transplant who was admitted with fever, right hemiparesis, slowness of speech, and difficulty in swallowing. (*A, B*) Axial T2-weighted images demonstrate multifocal hyperintense lesions in the bilateral cerebral hemispheres and upper brainstem. (*C, D*) Axial and coronal postcontrast T1-weighted images illustrate patchy enhancement, neither masslike nor ring enhancing, suggestive of cerebritis or encephalitis in an immunocompromised patient. (*E*) Gross photograph shows radiologic-pathologic correlation for the largest lesion in the left frontal lobe. (*F*) Hematoxylin-eosin stain photomicrograph reveals amastigote forms of *Trypanosoma cruzi* within macrophages (eg, bottom center). Reactivation of chronic Chagas disease can cause meningoencephalitis or brain abscesses (chagomas).

with heterogeneous enhancement and possible infarcts or hemorrhage related to the necrotizing angitis.[35,36] Diagnosis is confirmed by biopsy and histologic confirmation of trophozoites; screening multiplex polymerase chain reaction (PCR) of the CSF is highly specific and takes less than 5 hours but is not widely available.[37]

VIRAL LESIONS

In 1981, AIDS was first clinically observed in clusters of homosexual men with *Pneumocystis* pneumonia or Kaposi sarcoma. In 1983, Françoise Barré-Sinoussi and Luc Montagnier isolated and described the underlying pathogen, for which they received the 2008 Nobel Prize in Physiology or Medicine.[38] HIV, the first known lentivirus, infects and destroys CD4+ T lymphocytes, the regulators (helper cells) of the adaptive immune systems.

In addition to causing AIDS (CD4 count <200 cells/mm³) and, therefore, opportunistic infections/cancers, it can directly affect the nervous system, primarily via microglial cells. As expected, the prevalence of both HIV-associated dementia and HIV-associated distal sensory polyneuropathy declined after introduction of HAART in 1996.[39] On imaging, HIV-associated dementia causes symmetric nonenhancing T2/fluid-attenuated inversion recovery (FLAIR) hyperintense gliosis with volume loss in the periventricular and deep white matter; other names for this presentation include HIV encephalitis and AIDS dementia complex.[19,40]

The most frequent CNS opportunistic infections in AIDS patients remain the same in the HAART era: tuberculosis (bacteria), cryptococcosis (fungus), toxoplasmosis (parasite), and progressive multifocal leukoencephalopathy (PML) (virus).[41] PML is caused by JC virus, which is a common human polyomavirus. Most individuals undergo an asymptomatic primary infection during childhood; in one study, 86% of healthy adults were seropositive for antibodies to JC virus (100% of PML patients).[42] T-cell deficiency from AIDS or immunosuppressive medications (eg, natalizumab) allows the latent JC virus to reactivate and infect oligodendrocytes in the CNS, causing demyelinating lesions that coalesce and involve the subcortical U-fibers, with restricted diffusion at the margins due to swollen cells (**Fig. 8**). In classic PML, there is little edema or enhancement; inflammatory PML is usually seen in the setting of HAART and immune reconstitution inflammatory syndrome, although it can also be seen de novo in non-HIV patients.[43,44]

Herpesviridae is a family of DNA viruses that cause latent infections in animals. There are 8 human herpesviruses (HHVs). Herpes simplex virus 1 and herpes simplex virus 2 (also known as HHV-1 and HHV-2) cause orolabial and genital lesions; they also can cause encephalitis in both the immunocompetent and the immunocompromised. There is a predilection for the temporal lobes and limbic system, but disease may be more extensive in the immunocompromised (eg, brainstem involvement).[40,45] Rapid empiric therapy with IV acyclovir is critical; mortality rate exceeds 70% with inadequate treatment. Varicella zoster virus

(HHV-3) can also reactivate and cause encephalitis or myelitis, specifically due to vasculitis that involves large vessels in the immunocompetent and small vessels in the immunocompromised.[46] Cytomegalovirus (HHV-5) can cause opportunistic ventriculoencephalitis; imaging findings may be subtle or absent.[47,48]

NEOPLASTIC LESIONS

Viruses may indirectly or directly contribute to tumor development and are responsible for 15% of total cancer incidence (second only to tobacco use).[49] Two HHVs have demonstrated oncogenic potential: Epstein-Barr virus (EBV) (HHV-4) and Kaposi sarcoma–associated herpesvirus (HHV-8). The exact mechanism by which EBV is able to induce Burkitt lymphoma, nasopharyngeal carcinoma, or other lymphoproliferative disease remains unclear. Under the 2016 World Health Organization CNS classification, a subcategory of immunodeficiency-associated CNS lymphoma includes AIDS-related or EBV-positive diffuse

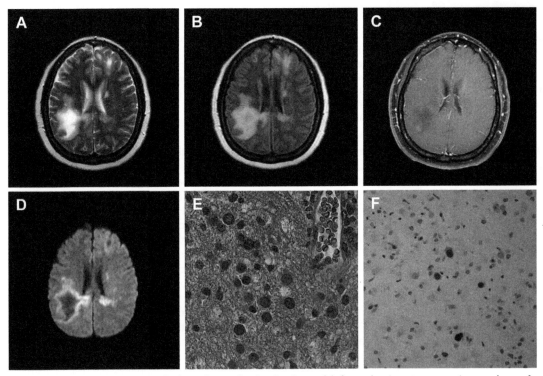

Fig. 8. A 53-year-old woman with slurred speech, dysphagia, and left-predominant progressive weakness for 2 weeks. Her laboratory tests revealed HIV positivity with a viral load of 59,800 and a CD4 count of 32. (*A–C*) Axial T2-weighted, T2-weighted FLAIR, and postcontrast T1-weighted images show asymmetric confluent T2 hyperintense lesions in the cerebral white matter, with peripheral involvement of subcortical U-fibers and without significant mass effect or enhancement. (*D*) Axial diffusion-weighted imaging demonstrates restricted diffusion at the lesion margins due to swollen oligodendrocytes. (*E*) Hematoxylin-eosin stain photomicrograph reveals oligodendrocytes with intranuclear viral inclusions on the left plus perivascular inflammation in the upper right. (*F*) SV40 immunohistochemical stain is cross-reactive for JC virus and confirms a diagnosis of PML.

large B-cell lymphoma (a subtype of primary CNS lymphoma [PCNSL]) and lymphomatoid granulomatosis (a rare EBV-driven angiocentric lymphoproliferative process that can affect the lungs and CNS).[50,51] Detection of EBV DNA in the CSF using either singleplex or multiplex PCR may help in the differential diagnosis of CNS lymphoma versus opportunistic infection but does not replace gold-standard biopsies or cultures.[52,53]

Tumor cells in immunodeficiency-associated CNS lymphoma (eg, AIDS and post-transplant) are positive for EBV-encoded RNA (EBER) in more than 90% of cases.[54,55] Similar to nonimmunodeficiency or EBV-negative diffuse large B-cell lymphoma, there is angiocentric proliferation of large atypical lymphocytes; high cellular density correlates with hyperattenuation on CT and low T2/apparent diffusion coefficient signal on MR imaging. There are a few important differences: immunocompetent PCNSL is unifocal in two-thirds of cases and typically homogeneously enhancing (non-necrotic); immunodeficient PCNSL is multifocal in two-thirds of cases and

typically ring enhancing (from necrosis) or nonenhancing (**Fig. 9**).[56,57] Ring-enhancing lesions with central restricted diffusion can be seen in pyogenic, tuberculous, or fungal abscesses; ringenhancing lesions without central restricted diffusion can be seen in toxoplasmic encephalitis or EBV-associated PCNSL. Associated hypermetabolism on thallium-201 single-photon emission CT or fluorodeoxyglucose PET supports the latter diagnosis.[58]

In 1970, an association between leiomyosarcoma and immunosuppression was first described. In 1995, 2 simultaneous publications found a link to EBV in both AIDS and post-transplant patients.[59–61] EBV-associated smooth muscle tumor (EBV-SMT) has since been reported in multiple organ systems, with locations in CNS, soft tissue, and lung accounting for roughly half of total cases; level of mitotic activity is the most dependable prognostic indicator.[62] In the CNS, they usually present as enhancing dural-based masses (**Fig. 10**), although there is 1 case report of an intra-axial EBV-SMT in the basal ganglia.[63,64] Many patients

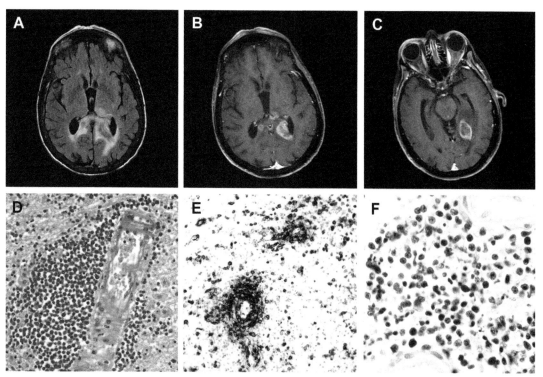

Fig. 9. An 85-year-old woman on mycophenolate mofetil for amyopathic dermatomyositis status post fall with abnormal findings on outside head CT. She also reports progressive memory deficits over the past year. (A) Axial T2-weighted FLAIR images shows edema in the periatrial regions, left greater than right, involving the splenium and left thalamus. (B, C) Axial postcontrast T1-weighted images reveal ring-enhancing lesions near the margins of the lateral ventricles, left greater than right. Primary concern was for immunodeficiency-associated CNS lymphoma, which was confirmed by a stereotactic needle biopsy. (D) Hematoxylin-eosin stain photomicrograph depicts cuffing of small round blue cells (B lymphocytes) around blood vessels. (E, F) Immunohistochemical stains for CD20 (B-cell marker) and EBER are both positive.

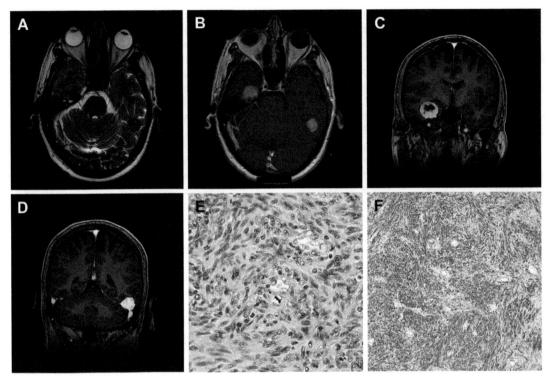

Fig. 10. A 46-year-old man with history of HIV/AIDS and disseminated histoplasmosis 1 year prior has new right-sided hearing loss and dizziness. (*A, B*) Axial T2-weighted and postcontrast T1-weighted images reveal enhancing T2 hypointense masses in both right anterior and left posterior temporal regions. (*C, D*) Coronal postcontrast T1-weighted images confirm their extra-axial dural-based location. Given the past medical history, granulomatous disease (eg, histoplasmosis) is a reasonable consideration. (*E*) Hematoxylin-eosin stain photomicrograph demonstrates a nonspecific spindle cell lesion (storiform and fascicular pattern) with a mitotic figure near the center. (*F*) Immunohistochemical stain for muscle-specific actin is positive, and in situ hybridization for EBER also is positive (not shown), consistent with EBV-SMT.

have multiple tumors, which reflect multiple infection events not metastases (clonally distinct).[65] Radiologic differential diagnosis includes meningiomas, metastases, and granulomas.[66] For a spindle cell lesion in an immunocompromised patient, pathologic differential diagnosis includes Kaposi sarcoma (positive endothelial markers) and mycobacterial spindle cell pseudotumor (acid-fast bacilli).[67]

SUMMARY

As discussed previously, the innate and adaptive immune systems are responsible for defending the bodies through a continuous process of detecting and destroying foreign or abnormal cells. Congenital or acquired defects in physical barriers, humoral immunity, or cellular immunity increase the risk of opportunistic infections and neoplasms, many of which affect the CNS and cause significant morbidity in the immunocompromised. For example, ring-enhancing lesions with central restricted diffusion can be seen in pyogenic,

tuberculous, or fungal abscesses; ring-enhancing lesions without central restricted diffusion can be seen in toxoplasmic encephalitis or EBV-associated PCNSL. Recognition of these and other neuroimaging patterns can help narrow the differential diagnosis, although in most cases a definitive diagnosis is established by clinical or anatomic pathology, utilizing serology, CSF PCR (either singleplex or multiplex), and cultures or biopsies.

REFERENCES

1. Litman GW, Cannon JP, Dishaw LJ. Reconstructing immune phylogeny: new perspectives. Nat Rev Immunol 2005;5(11):866–79.
2. Cunha BA. Central nervous system infections in the compromised host: a diagnostic approach. Infect Dis Clin North Am 2001;15(2):567–90.
3. Pruitt AA. Central nervous system infections complicating immunosuppression and transplantation. Continuum (Minneap Minn) 2018;24(5, Neuroinfectious Disease):1370–96.

4. Kemper AR, Davis MM, Freed GL. Expected adverse events in mass smallpox vaccination campaign. Eff Clin Pract 2002;5(2):84–90.

5. The Nobel prize in physiology or medicine 2018. NobelPrize.org. Nobel Media AB 2019. Available at: https://www.nobelprize.org/prizes/medicine/2018/summary/. Accessed July 31, 2019.

6. Shih RY, Koeller KK. Bacterial, fungal, and parasitic infections of the central nervous system: radiologic-pathologic correlation and historical perspectives. Radiographics 2015;35(4):1141–69.

7. Thigpen MC, Whitney CG, Messonnier NE, et al. Bacterial meningitis in the United States, 1998-2007. N Engl J Med 2011;364(21):2016–25.

8. Smith CIE, Berglöf A. X-Linked Agammaglobulinemia. In: Adam MP, Ardinger HH, Pagon RA, et al, editors. GeneReviews [Internet]. Seattle (WA): University of Washington, Seattle; 1993-2019. Available at: https://www.ncbi.nlm.nih.gov/books/NBK1453/.

9. Dionne B, Dehority W, Brett M, et al. The asplenic patient: post-insult immunocompetence, infection, and vaccination. Surg Infect (Larchmt) 2017;18(5):536–44.

10. Tunkel AR, Hartman BJ, Kaplan SL, et al. Practice guidelines for the management of bacterial meningitis. Clin Infect Dis 2004;39(9):1267–84.

11. Enzmann DR, Britt RH, Placone R. Staging of human brain abscess by computed tomography. Radiology 1983;146(3):703–8.

12. Enzmann DR, Brant-Zawadzki M, Britt RH. CT of central nervous system infections in immunocompromised patients. AJR Am J Roentgenol 1980;135(2):263–7.

13. Tilney LG, Portnoy DA. Actin filaments and the growth, movement, and spread of the intracellular bacterial parasite, Listeria monocytogenes. J Cell Biol 1989;109(4 Pt 1):1597–608.

14. Schuchat A, Deaver KA, Wenger JD, et al. Role of foods in sporadic listeriosis. I. Case-control study of dietary risk factors. The Listeria Study Group. JAMA 1992;267(15):2041–5.

15. Alper G, Knepper L, Kanal E. MR findings in listerial rhombencephalitis. AJNR Am J Neuroradiol 1996;17(3):593–6.

16. Campos LG, Trindade RA, Faistauer Â, et al. Rhombencephalitis: pictorial essay. Radiol Bras 2016;49(5):329–36.

17. Patkar D, Narang J, Yanamandala R, et al. Central nervous system tuberculosis: pathophysiology and imaging findings. Neuroimaging Clin N Am 2012;22(4):677–705.

18. Zakaria A, Elwatidy S, Elgamal E. Nocardia brain abscess: severe CNS infection that needs aggressive management; case report. Acta Neurochir (Wien) 2008;150(10):1097–101.

19. Smith AB, Smirniotopoulos JG, Rushing EJ. From the archives of the AFIP: central nervous system infections associated with human immunodeficiency virus infection: radiologic-pathologic correlation. Radiographics 2008;28(7):2033–58.

20. Starkey J, Moritani T, Kirby P. MRI of CNS fungal infections: review of aspergillosis to histoplasmosis and everything in between. Clin Neuroradiol 2014;24(3):217–30.

21. Berkefeld J, Enzensberger W, Lanfermann H. Cryptococcus meningoencephalitis in AIDS: parenchymal and meningeal forms. Neuroradiology 1999;41(2):129–33.

22. Lai PH, Lin SM, Pan HB, et al. Disseminated miliary cerebral candidiasis. AJNR Am J Neuroradiol 1997;18(7):1303–6.

23. Sonneville R, Magalhaes E, Meyfroidt G. Central nervous system infections in immunocompromised patients. Curr Opin Crit Care 2017;23(2):128–33.

24. Castro I, Ruiz J, Tasias M, et al. Central nervous system infections in immunocompromised patients. Rev Esp Quimioter 2018;31(Suppl 1):56–61.

25. Ashdown BC, Tien RD, Felsberg GJ. Aspergillosis of the brain and paranasal sinuses in immunocompromised patients: CT and MR imaging findings. AJR Am J Roentgenol 1994;162(1):155–9.

26. Charlot M, Pialat JB, Obadia N, et al. Diffusion-weighted imaging in brain aspergillosis. Eur J Neurol 2007;14(8):912–6.

27. Herrera DA, Dublin AB, Ormsby EL, et al. Imaging findings of rhinocerebral mucormycosis. Skull Base 2009;19(2):117–25.

28. Lammering JC, Iv M, Gupta N, et al. Imaging spectrum of CNS coccidioidomycosis: prevalence and significance of concurrent brain and spinal disease. AJR Am J Roentgenol 2013;200(6):1334–46.

29. Walker M, Zunt JR. Parasitic central nervous system infections in immunocompromised hosts. Clin Infect Dis 2005;40(7):1005–15.

30. Jones JL, Roberts JM. Toxoplasmosis hospitalizations in the United States, 2008, and trends, 1993-2008. Clin Infect Dis 2012;54(7):e58–61.

31. Dubey JP, Lindsay DS, Speer CA. Structures of Toxoplasma gondii tachyzoites, bradyzoites, and sporozoites and biology and development of tissue cysts. Clin Microbiol Rev 1998;11(2):267–99.

32. Sugden K, Moffitt TE, Pinto L, et al. Is toxoplasma gondii infection related to brain and behavior impairments in humans? evidence from a population-representative birth cohort. PLoS One 2016;11(2):e0148435.

33. Lee GT, Antelo F, Mlikotic AA. Best cases from the AFIP: cerebral toxoplasmosis. Radiographics 2009;29(4):1200–5.

34. Kumar GG, Mahadevan A, Guruprasad AS, et al. Eccentric target sign in cerebral toxoplasmosis: neuropathological correlate to the imaging feature. J Magn Reson Imaging 2010;31(6):1469–72.

35. Schumacher DJ, Tien RD, Lane K. Neuroimaging findings in rare amebic infections of the central nervous system. AJNR Am J Neuroradiol 1995;16(4 Suppl):930–5.

36. Singh P, Kochhar R, Vashishta RK, et al. Amebic meningoencephalitis: spectrum of imaging findings. AJNR Am J Neuroradiol 2006;27(6):1217–21.

37. Qvarnstrom Y, Visvesvara GS, Sriram R, et al. Multiplex real-time PCR assay for simultaneous detection of Acanthamoeba spp., Balamuthia mandrillaris, and Naegleria fowleri. J Clin Microbiol 2006;44(10): 3589–95.

38. Barré-Sinoussi F, Chermann JC, Rey F, et al. Isolation of a T-lymphotropic retrovirus from a patient at risk for acquired immune deficiency syndrome (AIDS). Science 1983;220(4599):868–71.

39. Maschke M, Kastrup O, Esser S, et al. Incidence and prevalence of neurological disorders associated with HIV since the introduction of highly active antiretroviral therapy (HAART). J Neurol Neurosurg Psychiatry 2000;69(3):376–80.

40. Koeller KK, Shih RY. Viral and prion infections of the central nervous system: radiologic-pathologic correlation: from the radiologic pathology archives. Radiographics 2017;37(1):199–233.

41. Manzardo C, Del Mar Ortega M, Sued O, et al. Central nervous system opportunistic infections in developed countries in the highly active antiretroviral therapy era. J Neurovirol 2005;11(Suppl 3): 72–82.

42. Weber T, Trebst C, Frye S, et al. Analysis of the systemic and intrathecal humoral immune response in progressive multifocal leukoencephalopathy. J Infect Dis 1997;176(1):250–4.

43. Sarbu N, Shih RY, Jones RV, et al. White matter diseases with radiologic-pathologic correlation. Radiographics 2016;36(5):1426–47.

44. Bag AK, Curé JK, Chapman PR, et al. JC virus infection of the brain. AJNR Am J Neuroradiol 2010;31(9): 1564–76.

45. Bulakbasi N, Kocaoglu M. Central nervous system infections of herpesvirus family. Neuroimaging Clin N Am 2008;18(1):53–84.

46. Chiang F, Panyaping T, Tedesqui G, et al. Varicella zoster CNS vascular complications. A report of four cases and literature review. Neuroradiol J 2014;27(3):327–33.

47. Post MJ, Hensley GT, Moskowitz LB, et al. Cytomegalic inclusion virus encephalitis in patients with AIDS: CT, clinical, and pathologic correlation. AJR Am J Roentgenol 1986;146(6):1229–34.

48. Clifford DB, Arribas JR, Storch GA, et al. Magnetic resonance brain imaging lacks sensitivity for AIDS associated cytomegalovirus encephalitis. J Neurovirol 1996;2(6):397–403.

49. zur Hausen H. Viruses in human cancers. Science 1991;254(5035):1167–73.

50. Louis DN, Perry A, Reifenberger G, et al. The 2016 World Health Organization classification of tumors of the central nervous system: a summary. Acta Neuropathol 2016;131(6):803–20.

51. Koeller KK, Shih RY. Extranodal lymphoma of the central nervous system and spine. Radiol Clin North Am 2016;54(4):649–71.

52. Arribas JR, Clifford DB, Fichtenbaum CJ, et al. Detection of epstein-barr virus DNA in cerebrospinal fluid for diagnosis of AIDS-related central nervous system lymphoma. J Clin Microbiol 1995;33(6):1580–3.

53. Rhein J, Bahr NC, Hemmert AC, et al. Diagnostic performance of a multiplex PCR assay for meningitis in an HIV-infected population in Uganda. Diagn Microbiol Infect Dis 2016;84(3):268–73.

54. Bibas M, Antinori A. EBV and HIV-related lymphoma. Mediterr J Hematol Infect Dis 2009;1(2): e2009032.

55. Chou AP, Lalezari S, Fong BM, et al. Post-transplantation primary central nervous system lymphoma: a case report and review of the literature. Surg Neurol Int 2011;2:130.

56. Küker W, Nägele T, Korfel A, et al. Primary central nervous system lymphomas (PCNSL): MRI features at presentation in 100 patients. J Neurooncol 2005; 72(2):169–77.

57. Thurnher MM, Rieger A, Kleibl-Popov C, et al. Primary central nervous system lymphoma in AIDS: a wider spectrum of CT and MRI findings. Neuroradiology 2001;43(1):29–35.

58. Haldorsen IS, Espeland A, Larsson EM. Central nervous system lymphoma: characteristic findings on traditional and advanced imaging. AJNR Am J Neuroradiol 2011;32(6):984–92.

59. Pritzker KP, Huang SN, Marshall KG. Malignant tumours following immunosuppressive therapy. Can Med Assoc J 1970;103(13):1362–5.

60. McClain KL, Leach CT, Jenson HB, et al. Association of Epstein-Barr virus with leiomyosarcomas in young people with AIDS. N Engl J Med 1995; 332(1):12–8.

61. Lee ES, Locker J, Nalesnik M, et al. The association of Epstein-Barr virus with smooth-muscle tumors occurring after organ transplantation. N Engl J Med 1995;332(1):19–25.

62. Purgina B, Rao UN, Miettinen M, et al. AIDS-related EBV-associated smooth muscle tumors: a review of 64 published cases. Patholog Res Int 2011;2011: 561548.

63. Lohan R, Bathla G, Gupta S, et al. Epstein-Barr virus (EBV)-related smooth muscle tumors of central nervous system–a report of two cases and review of literature. Clin Imaging 2013; 37(3):564–8.

64. Kumar S, Santi M, Vezina G, et al. Epstein-Barr virus-associated smooth muscle tumor of the basal ganglia in an HIV+ child: case report and review

of the literature. Pediatr Dev Pathol 2004;7(2): 198–203.

65. Deyrup AT, Lee VK, Hill CE, et al. Epstein-Barr virus-associated smooth muscle tumors are distinctive mesenchymal tumors reflecting multiple infection events: a clinicopathologic and molecular analysis of 29 tumors from 19 patients. Am J Surg Pathol 2006;30(1):75–82.

66. Smith AB, Horkanyne-Szakaly I, Schroeder JW, et al. From the radiologic pathology archives: mass lesions of the dura: beyond meningioma-radiologic-pathologic correlation. Radiographics 2014;34(2): 295–312.

67. Dekate J, Chetty R. Epstein-barr virus-associated smooth muscle tumor. Arch Pathol Lab Med 2016; 140(7):718–22.

UNITED STATES POSTAL SERVICE®

Statement of Ownership, Management, and Circulation (All Periodicals Publications Except Requester Publications)

1. Publication Title	2. Publication Number	3. Filing Date
RADIOLOGIC CLINICS OF NORTH AMERICA	596 – 510	9/18/2019

4. Issue Frequency	5. Number of Issues Published Annually	6. Annual Subscription Price
JAN, MAR, MAY, JUL, SEP, NOV	6	$508.00

7. Complete Mailing Address of Known Office of Publication (Not printer) (Street, city, county, state, and ZIP+4®)

ELSEVIER INC.
230 Park Avenue, Suite 800
New York, NY 10169

Contact Person
STEPHEN R. BUSHING

Telephone (Include area code)
215-239-3688

8. Complete Mailing Address of Headquarters or General Business Office of Publisher (Not printer)

ELSEVIER INC.
230 Park Avenue, Suite 800
New York, NY 10169

9. Full Names and Complete Mailing Addresses of Publisher, Editor, and Managing Editor (Do not leave blank)

Publisher (Name and complete mailing address)

TAYLOR BALL, ELSEVIER INC.
1600 JOHN F KENNEDY BLVD. SUITE 1800
PHILADELPHIA, PA 19103-2899

Editor (Name and complete mailing address)

JOHN VASSALLO, ELSEVIER INC.
1600 JOHN F KENNEDY BLVD. SUITE 1800
PHILADELPHIA, PA 19103-2899

Managing Editor (Name and complete mailing address)

PATRICK MANLEY, ELSEVIER INC.
1600 JOHN F KENNEDY BLVD. SUITE 1800
PHILADELPHIA, PA 19103-2899

10. Owner (Do not leave blank. If the publication is owned by a corporation, give the name and address of the corporation immediately followed by the names and addresses of all stockholders owning or holding 1 percent or more of the total amount of stock. If not owned by a corporation, give the names and addresses of the individual owners. If owned by a partnership or other unincorporated firm, give its name and address as well as those of each individual owner. If the publication is published by a nonprofit organization, give its name and address.)

Full Name	Complete Mailing Address
WHOLLY OWNED SUBSIDIARY OF REED/ELSEVIER, US HOLDINGS	1600 JOHN F KENNEDY BLVD. SUITE 1800 PHILADELPHIA, PA 19103-2899

11. Known Bondholders, Mortgagees, and Other Security Holders Owning or Holding 1 Percent or More of Total Amount of Bonds, Mortgages, or Other Securities. If none, check box ▶ ☐ None

Full Name	Complete Mailing Address
N/A	

12. Tax Status (For completion by nonprofit organizations authorized to mail at nonprofit rates) (Check one)
The purpose, function, and nonprofit status of this organization and the exempt status for federal income tax purposes:
☒ Has Not Changed During Preceding 12 Months
☐ Has Changed During Preceding 12 Months (Publisher must submit explanation of change with this statement)

PS Form 3526, July 2014 [Page 1 of 4 (see instructions page 4)]   PSN: 7530-01-000-9631   PRIVACY NOTICE: See our privacy policy on www.usps.com.

---

13. Publication Title	14. Issue Date for Circulation Data Below
RADIOLOGIC CLINICS OF NORTH AMERICA	JULY 2019

15. Extent and Nature of Circulation

		Average No. Copies Each Issue During Preceding 12 Months	No. Copies of Single Issue Published Nearest to Filing Date
a. Total Number of Copies (Net press run)		767	911
b. Paid Circulation (By Mail and Outside the Mail)	(1) Mailed Outside-County Paid Subscriptions Stated on PS Form 3541 (Include paid distribution above nominal rate, advertiser's proof copies, and exchange copies)	502	615
	(2) Mailed In-County Paid Subscriptions Stated on PS Form 3541 (Include paid distribution above nominal rate, advertiser's proof copies, and exchange copies)	0	0
	(3) Paid Distribution Outside the Mails Including Sales Through Dealers and Carriers, Street Vendors, Counter Sales, and Other Paid Distribution Outside USPS®	176	249
	(4) Paid Distribution by Other Classes of Mail Through the USPS (e.g., First-Class Mail®)	0	0
c. Total Paid Distribution (Sum of 15b (1), (2), (3), and (4))	▶	678	864
d. Free or Nominal Rate Distribution (By Mail and Outside the Mail)	(1) Free or Nominal Rate Outside-County Copies Included on PS Form 3541	74	30
	(2) Free or Nominal Rate In-County Copies Included on PS Form 3541	0	0
	(3) Free or Nominal Rate Copies Mailed at Other Classes Through the USPS (e.g., First-Class Mail)	0	0
	(4) Free or Nominal Rate Distribution Outside the Mail (Carriers or other means)	74	30
e. Total Free or Nominal Rate Distribution (Sum of 15d (1), (2), (3) and (4))	▶	74	30
f. Total Distribution (Sum of 15c and 15e)	▶	752	894
g. Copies not Distributed (See Instructions to Publishers #4 (page #3))	▶	15	17
h. Total (Sum of 15f and g)	▶	767	911
i. Percent Paid (15c divided by 15f times 100)		90.16%	96.64%

* If you are claiming electronic copies, go to line 16 on page 3. If you are not claiming electronic copies, skip to line 17 on page 3.

PS Form 3526, July 2014 (Page 2 of 4)

16. Electronic Copy Circulation

	Average No. Copies Each Issue During Preceding 12 Months	No. Copies of Single Issue Published Nearest to Filing Date
a. Paid Electronic Copies	▶	
b. Total Paid Print Copies (Line 15c) + Paid Electronic Copies (Line 16a)	▶	
c. Total Print Distribution (Line 15f) + Paid Electronic Copies (Line 16a)	▶	
d. Percent Paid (Both Print & Electronic Copies) (16b divided by 16c × 100)	▶	

☒ I certify that 50% of all my distributed copies (electronic and print) are paid above a nominal price.

17. Publication of Statement of Ownership

☒ If the publication is a general publication, publication of this statement is required. Will be printed in the NOVEMBER 2019 issue of this publication.   ☐ Publication not required.

18. Signature and Title of Editor, Publisher, Business Manager, or Owner

STEPHEN R. BUSHING - INVENTORY DISTRIBUTION CONTROL MANAGER

Date 9/18/2019

I certify that all information furnished on this form is true and complete. I understand that anyone who furnishes false or misleading information on this form or who omits material or information requested on the form may be subject to criminal sanctions (including fines and imprisonment) and/or civil sanctions (including civil penalties).

PS Form 3526, July 2014 (Page 3 of 4)   PRIVACY NOTICE: See our privacy policy on www.usps.com

Printed and bound by CPI Group (UK) Ltd, Croydon, CR0 4YY

08/05/2025

01864747-0015